Contents

"Highly recommend Reflexology
for Babies and Children. Sue's gentle
touch approach is simple, helpful
and fun to do!

This well written and beautifully
illustrated book is the first of of it's
kind and is a complete resource for
anyone interested in babies!"

Michelle Emanuel
Occupational Therapist, CranioSacral Therapist,
Certified Infant Massage Instructor,
Cincinnati, OH, USA

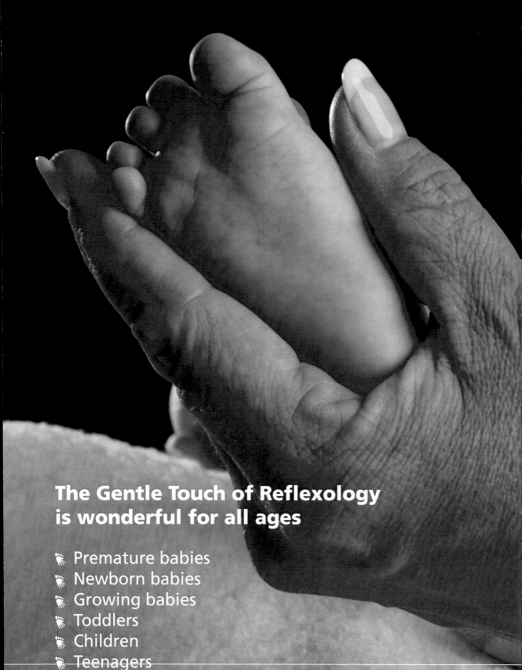

The Gentle Touch of Reflexology is wonderful for all ages

- Premature babies
- Newborn babies
- Growing babies
- Toddlers
- Children
- Teenagers

Introduction

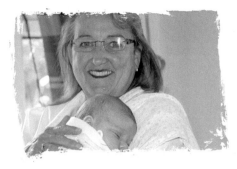

This book has been written to meet the needs of a diverse readership.
I recognise that you (the reader) may be reading this for various reasons.

The book will be useful to you if:

- You are a practitioner of Reflexology and wish to learn more about how to work with and treat babies and children
- You are interested in and want to know more about how Reflexology can help the younger generation
- You have children or grandchildren and want to know how Reflexology might help
- You are practising or studying Gentle Touch™ Reflexology

This book will provide you with:

- A treatment routine plus information on how to treat babies and children
- Information on common ailments and conditions
- Knowledge on how to create a suitable treatment for each child
- An overview of factors that are worth considering regarding the health and happiness of both babies and children

I have endeavoured to keep the language straight forward, easy to understand and relevant, whilst also being both instructive and informative.

The book can be read from beginning to end so that you can follow the flow of the text. I have written it so that each section can be read in isolation. You can therefore, dip in and out as you require, according to your area(s) of interest. I will take you through considerations that I have personally found to be useful when working with babies and children.

The content is relevant to both parents and Reflexologists. However, some sections are specific to Reflexology Practitioners and these have been highlighted in Deep Purple and marked with a Practitioner symbol to make them easier to identify.

Reflexology for Babies and Children

The benefits of Reflexology for both babies and children are endless and, although sometimes underestimated, this wonderfully simple and effective therapy can be perfect for them. Amongst the many reasons why this therapy is so helpful, supportive and healing for the younger generation are that it can help them to become more confident, improve their sleep, reduce irritability or relieve physical discomfort.

Reflexology is as suitable for a tiny baby as it is for a child or an adult. There are now children's charities, organisations, schools and even doctors offering Reflexology for their young clients. This is wonderful news for all the babies and children who will benefit from Reflexology in their younger years and take this advantage into adulthood. Everyone wins!

Our children are our future. If we can offer Reflexology as a support / pick me up or solution provider, then we help them towards a better life.

Why Reflexology?

The ancient art of Reflexology has been used by many cultures for centuries. There are references going back to the time of the ancient Egyptians, early Europeans and even past American presidents. It is still used in many eastern countries in open air or ad-hoc locations. All the depictions, engravings and photographs show only adults having Reflexology. There is, however, a real and valuable place for Reflexology for our younger generation too.

More families are starting to take greater responsibility for their own health. It is now much more acceptable to take a child for treatments to a complementary practitioner. My own experiences in clinic have shown me that my younger clients usually come along following a personal recommendation from an adult who has had some successful treatment, and wants the same for their child, grandchild or friend's child. It is good to see the increasing number of organisations that wish to introduce the treatment of Reflexology into the list of services on offer. I am delighted that it is now becoming a much more freely accepted and requested form of treatment.

What is Reflexology?

Reflexology is the massage and application of touch to a specific area of the foot, or hand. Every area of the body has an associated reflex point on the foot that reflects the condition of an individual area, organ or system of the body. There are many different forms of Reflexology and they vary in style and pressure. All forms of Reflexology, however, offer some lovely outcomes. This book specifically deals with Gentle Touch™ Reflexology which is one form of Reflexology that is especially suited to both babies and children.

Gentle Touch™ Reflexology can be done on either the hands or the feet and is suitable for all ages. It is the very lightness of touch that makes it so suitable for the youngest of children and throughout their lives. The therapeutic touch applied to certain parts of either the hands or feet can have an effect on certain parts of their body or the whole child. The light touch or massage is applied to the areas known as reflex points. It is the correct working of these points that has been found to have a significant benefit. Gentle Touch™ Reflexology is a wonderful treatment and is both pleasurable to give and to receive.

History of Reflexology

The practice of Reflexology is nothing new. It has been practised by many of the ancient cultures, including the Chinese, Egyptians, North American Indians and Aboriginals. The ancient Egyptians even had a carving on the wall of the tomb of physician Ankhmahor at Saggara, Egypt.

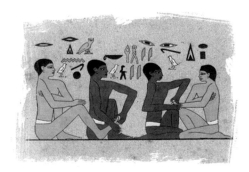

In the early 1900's Dr William Fitzgerald - an American Ear, Nose and Throat Surgeon from Connecticut discovered that, by using pressure on the feet, he could produce a kind of anaesthetising effect on his patients. He published his findings in a book called Zone Therapy.

Dr Joseph Shelby Riley and his wife Elizabeth, were impressed by the therapy and theories, and attended one of Fitzgerald's courses. Dr Riley worked with Dr Fitzgerald and wrote numerous books on the subject of Reflexology. A qualified physiotherapist working with the Rileys', Eunice Ingham, used some body maps and ancient foot charts, that she found in the basement of a hospital, to locate all areas of the body on the feet. It was Eunice Ingham who devised the basic foot Reflexology map that is the basis of all charts used by reflexologists today.

Traditionally, Reflexology has always used varying amounts of heavy pressure, but, in modern times, this heavy pressure might not be as necessary. In years gone by people went about in bare feet or had poor footwear, so built up many more layers of hard skin to protect their feet and sustained a great deal more wear and tear than we do now. Today, we have thick shoes, soled slippers, thick carpets and cushioned underlay and therefore it is logical that we need less pressure to achieve not only the same but potentially better results. There is a great deal that can be achieved by working more sensitively. The Gentle Touch™ approach of Reflexology stems from the basic requirement to work with both adults, children and babies in the most sympathetic and sensitive way.

Relief from Constant Crying

"We were at our friends for Sunday lunch when my son was just weeks old. He cried constantly and nothing we did seemed to help. A few minutes of Reflexology from our friend worked wonders. I have never seen him relax so quickly and before you knew it – he was asleep. It seemed miraculous to me!"

Father R

The Beginning for Me

"If you rub their feet it sometimes brings them on"

Midwife

My own personal introduction to Reflexology was after my son was born in 1986. Both of us experienced a lengthy labour process and he was exhausted by the time he made his wonderful arrival. He was beautiful, tired and struggling to summon up the energy to feed. Everyone was a little concerned when he still could not feed the following day. Luckily a very loving and experienced midwife sat with us during the following night and told me that they have found that if you rub the soles of a baby's feet it sometimes 'brings them on!' I sat tenderly and patiently rubbing my son's feet and willing him to pick up enough energy to be able to feed (otherwise he would have to go down to the Special Care Baby Unit). I 'rubbed' his feet and he found the energy to feed!

My journey into working with babies and then children has mirrored my own life. When my sons were babies I found that Reflexology was superb for them. As they continued through into their childhoods, I ensured that they could always have treatments. It was really because of them that I started doing so much Reflexology for both babies and children. I treated my own, friend's and client's children. More and more children were coming to the clinic with every type of problem including:

- Earache
- 'Tummy' ache
- Poor sleeping habits
- Being agitated or hyperactive
- Lack of confidence
- Growing pains
- Exam stress
- Persistent coughs and colds

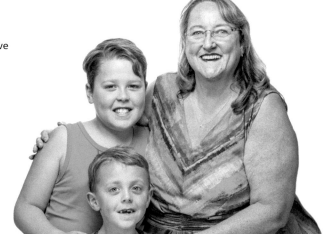

Why Reflexology is Helpful for Babies and Children

It can be amazing and gratifying to witness the support and assistance that Reflexology can offer for such a wide range of conditions and situations.

Babies

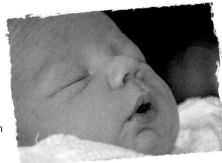

- Calming and relaxing
- Aids restful sleep
- Helps to boost their immune systems
- Improves digestive functions
- Helps to alleviate colic
- Can help to improve and maintain healthy skin
- Improves ability to breast-feed
- Improves bonding between Mother and Baby

Children

- Assists them to be or stay focused
- Improves concentration
- Improves ability to relax
- Improves and assists their immune system
- Improves self confidence and self esteem
- Helps to combat:
  - Headaches
  - 'Tummy' aches
  - Non-specific symptoms
  - Anxiety
  - Sleep disturbances
  - Hearing problems
  - Joint discomfort
  - Behavioural problems

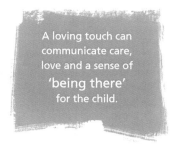

A loving touch can communicate care, love and a sense of **'being there'** for the child.

Note: The word 'children' relates to both younger and older children i.e. teenagers as well.

Miles of Smiles

It is delightful to see the impact that such a simple and yet effective treatment can have on a child that has been trying to cope with either a physical, emotional or an energetic challenge. You may see the effects during the treatment or it may become more obvious over time. It is common to see smiles, attention being paid to what you are doing or even just a simple comment of how it makes them feel. Children generally do not modify their responses and will regularly say it how it is; 'out of the mouth of babes'! If they say they like it or want a treatment again, it is probably because they really noticed the effect that it had, or liked the sensations that it generated.

Offering Added Value

There are many ways to assist children and their parents / guardians through Gentle Touch™ Reflexology and associated advice. Sometimes what makes the difference is:

- Purely a simple treatment
- A series of treatments
- A combination of the treatments and advice

Sometimes the treatment offered is only part of the value that the young person and their carer may receive. I started treating children when my own children were born and quickly realised that the treatments were invaluable for them. This is because they were both relaxing and provided a special time for them. This 'one to one' time may be one of the biggest assets in the treatment of children who are time starved or lack attention in general. Today's increasingly fast - paced world makes it harder to give the one to one attention that a child craves and requires. The combination of real attention paid throughout the treatment, together with some advice and guidance, can have a significant impact on a child's physical and emotional health.

"I love the reflexology treatments that we have. It is gentle, soothing and fabulous for rebalancing our energies. I can totally recommend it to anyone when any problems arise. It's totally safe and beautifully effective".

Dr Carolyn Eddleston, GP and Acupuncturist

Noticing the Three Potential Areas of Improvement

Gentle Touch™ Reflexology works on three levels:

- Physical
- Emotional
- Energetic

A child responds to treatments in many ways, although not necessarily in the way anticipated. It is possible that the child has a physical problem. After treatment the child could seem to be more relaxed and noticeably coping better with life. However, that was not the anticipated outcome, but it is a real benefit nevertheless. The improvement with the physical concern may follow later as the child's body may have internally prioritised that the emotional state of relaxation was the most important factor to be achieved and realised, before the physical issue could be addressed and resolved.

A person may want a specific outcome but other benefits may come first. The recipient of a Reflexology treatment may experience the benefits in any combination of physical, emotional or energetic improvements.

A balanced, healthy and happy child is a delight to have around. Reflexology can be one of the most soothing and enjoyable treatments that can assist a child towards achieving some, or all of these, potential improvements. Pay attention to all the improvements, even if they are not what you expected or planned!

"When You Take Hold of the Feet; You Take Hold of the Whole Person"

Being held is one of the most important factors for the healthy emotional and psychological growth of an individual. Gentle Touch™ Reflexology treatments can feel as if the person is 'being held', via the level of touch. We use a particular technique that is called the 'hug' or 'cuddle' (see page 78) as it can feel like a total hug, even though it is only directly experienced through the feet. If a child is really unwell or struggling emotionally then a simple gentle touch through the feet can have a deeply personal effect.

Some parents report that knowing how to do a few basic techniques can bring a form of emotional closeness that only a loving touch can convey. It may also be a child's way of asking for closeness as they request a treatment, or put their feet up on the parent's lap - a hint maybe?

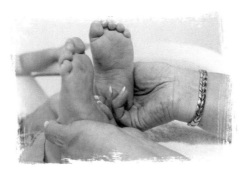

Touch

It is during the early, formative years that a child makes the first discoveries of their world, their body and what is happening around them. The joy of Gentle Touch™ Reflexology is that it is one way of introducing more appropriate touch for a child to enjoy, and continue to enjoy, as they grow up. It is an unfortunate fact that some children are touch deprived. This may be because the adult is too busy or too stressed to relax. Alternatively it maybe they find it too difficult to offer cuddles, hugs or mini massages as they were not used to it themselves. Reflexology can be something that fills the gap. This could be taking the child for treatments, or through learning a few simple techniques and using them within the family.

One of the most noticeable aspects of treating children is that they show their responses and attitudes quite freely. They are more responsive than adults who may have learnt to temper their responses according to current convention etc. Children, however, are more open in their responses. Children who have experienced Gentle Touch™ Reflexology will frequently ask for this lovely therapy and ask for "their feet to be rubbed", or say things like "do my feet please"! It helps children to be able to get their needs met, both physically and emotionally.

It is good to be able to offer a treatment that does not take long to do, has a 'magic touch', provides some 'one to one' attention and feels lovely as well. It is as sought after by healthy children as it is by children who are seriously ill or who have special needs.

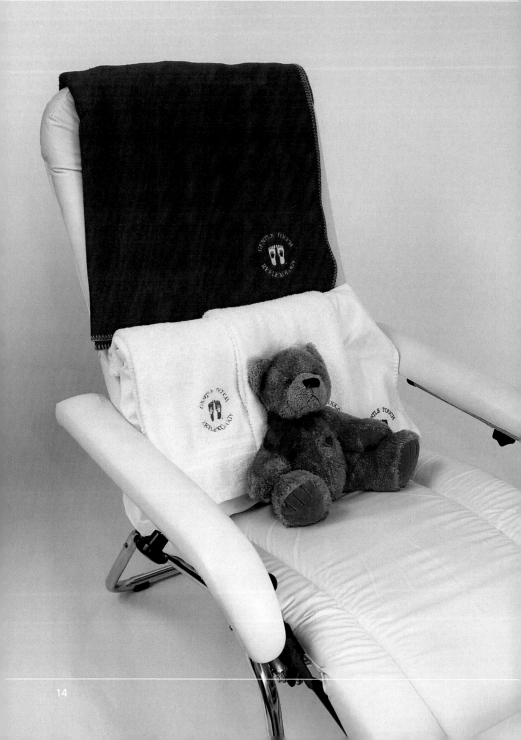

Treating a Child

Preparation Prior to Treating

Before you contemplate treating anyone of any age, it is essential that you pay attention to your own emotional, physical and mental state. Take a few minutes to prepare to treat and also 'ground' yourself. Imagine that you are in a beautiful breathable bubble and the chaos in the rest of the world is happening totally outside your bubble. This will give you a place in which to concentrate, relax and be completely focused on the child you are working on. It is also helpful to use a 'grounding' technique and imagine that your feet have tree roots that anchor you down through into the earth. This will help you to stay focused and safe.

- Remember to stay grounded
- Protect yourself with appropriate techniques
- Know what you like about yourself and the person that you are treating
- Focus on the child and not their condition or problem
- Focus on what is good and not what is wrong

The best treatments are conducted when the person doing the treatment is feeling safe, comfortable, grounded and relaxed. Energetically this is important too. You can use yoga, breathing, energy centering or one of the techniques that are detailed in full on my DVD's Energy Techniques and also Success Tips for Reflexologists.

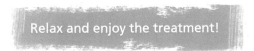

Relax and enjoy the treatment!

Energy Follows Thought

There are an increasing number of books currently available that remind us that what we think about is what we attract. We are becoming more comfortable in the message that "Energy follows thought". Therefore, if we focus on a condition then it is, in effect, making it more likely that the condition will continue or will return. The way forward is to recognise the gifts, joys, talents and potential of the child.

Remember to focus on the name of the person and who the person is.
An example is that it is better to treat 'Lucy' rather than 'the baby with colic'.
Pay attention to your own thoughts, your language and the language of anyone caring for the child.

I have expanded on the subject of 'energy follows thought' in my previous book, 'Three Steps to Enjoying Life'. (see www.suercks.com for more info)

Baby / Child or Condition?

You can treat a child to support their everyday life and enjoyment of life. You may also be treating a child because they are experiencing pain. This can lead to a common error as your focus may be on whatever they are suffering from, and not the actual child.

There can be a great deal of emotion around the condition, accident or symptoms of the baby or child. You may find yourself worrying or 'needing' to help the child overcome the illness or pain. It is essential to keep the prime focus on the child who is being treated and not the condition that they are experiencing. The results can be better and longer lasting when you focus on the child and the child's life rather than what is wrong with them.

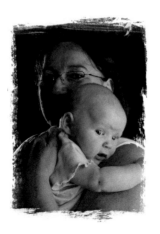

If you find yourself becoming caught up by the intensity of the emotion concerning the condition or illness of a child, it is helpful to redirect your thoughts towards another subject because 'energy follows thought'. When you notice that you are thinking about the child's colic or constipation (or any condition), change your thoughts to anything pleasant. This could be a countryside scene, a ball game, a pet, a holiday, their smile, when you last laughed - anything that is not 'constipation'!

It is really important to be aware of what you are thinking about. If you are thinking about their bouts of colic or constipation then you are inadvertently reducing the time that it might take for the child to recover. Whenever you treat and touch the reflex points you are doing this to assist the child and not change the condition. This can be hard in reality, as it is sometime difficult to forget the issue, and you may find yourself desperately hoping that this treatment may help. It is important to believe that you are going to do your best, not allow yourself to focus on the problem, and to treat to help the whole child. Reflexology is a holistic therapy, and works with the whole person assisting them to do their own healing from within.

Where to Treat

The best place to treat is anywhere that you and the child are comfortable. It is only possible to conduct a good, healthy and relaxing treatment if you are comfortable, as the treatment is so lovely, flowing and gentle. If you are uncomfortable it is hard to let the treatment flow, as your discomfort and tension will transmit through to the child. It is well worth working out what will be the best place for you to work, as well as where is practical for the child. If you wish to use reflexology for a child who is really sick in bed and you are extremely uncomfortable reaching over the end of the bed, then the treatment will not be as effective. When the setting is acceptable for both of you, then you can create the best opportunity for the highest level of treatment to be possible.

Take time to create the most pleasant atmosphere possible

- Comfortable temperature (not too hot or cold)
- Natural Light, (so it is easier to see the indications and changes)
- A private space where you are less likely to be interrupted
- Few distractions, therefore allowing both the child and person doing the treatment, an opportunity to focus and concentrate i.e. TV's, electronic games, lap tops etc. Consider what is appropriate for each situation as some children will only have a treatment if they are otherwise engaged by a game or another distraction. It is likely that over time, that less external stimulation will be required as they begin to notice the internal signals of comfort.

You can do treatments when:

- 🐾 The child is being held on someone else's knee
- 🐾 The child is lying in a cot or bed.
- 🐾 The child's feet are on your lap, or on a pillow on your knee.
- 🐾 The child sits in a recliner chair

Tiny babies can also be partially treated while you are holding them.

I recommended great flexibility when treating babies and children and if possible do the treatments where they are comfortable. Remember that you can treat on the beach, in the garden or anywhere whether it is inside or outside. As long as the child is happy with it and you are both comfortable, that's all that matters. Some of my most memorable treatments have been done outside as I am fortunate to be able to use my garden as an extra place to do treatments for my friends and their children.

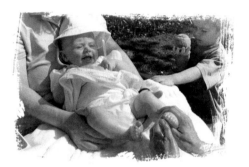

Safety is Paramount!

This brings us to an important issue of foot massage versus reflexology!
I defy any loving person who likes babies not to want to touch such gorgeous and cute feet. However, if you are a Reflexologist it brings into question whether you are just touching their feet or knowingly doing some Reflexology. You need to be mindful that whenever you hold a baby and touch their feet that it is just simple natural touch rather than 'Reflexology.' unless as a qualified Reflexologist, you have permission to treat (see Treatment Consent Form on page 28).

Hints for Set-Up Requirements when working with Babies and Children

When setting up to treat babies and children the following items are useful:

- Pillow / towels (a selection of sizes and thicknesses)
- Oil / lotion
- Tissues
- Non-toxic cleansing lotion
- Toys (distraction devices!)
- Books (for older children)
- Spare cloths (for babies and mopping up!)
- Somewhere comfortable for any accompanying adult to sit with the child or who may have the baby on their knee (depending on size)

Ensure all toys meet relevant child safety legislation and are thoroughly cleaned after use.

Always wash any towels at high temperature and as soon as possible after treatment. Do not leave towels ready for a big wash load as they need to be washed as soon as possible. This prevents contamination and also any staining from the use of oils etc.

Relief from Constipation

"My son had not filled his nappy (diaper) for three days and he was clearly very uncomfortable. Luckily we were going on holiday with my Mum who is a reflexologist. I asked her if she would treat him and she warned us that the result could be smelly! How right she was just as he had filled his nappy within two hours and then four more times in the next six!"

Father P

Respecting the Baby / Child's Responses

It is really important that everyone respects the needs and responses of all clients. That includes our youngest clients too. If a child is sick, they may wish to stay internally focused and not want to be 'messed about' by being treated. Interestingly, it may be precisely the soothing support of a treatment that helps. The only way to tell is to 'listen' to the response of the child.

There is a marked difference between lively and active movements when compared with movements indicating rejection of the treatment or touch. If they cry or pull away, this could be their only way to tell us if this treatment is not welcomed. Take time to notice and respect their wishes. Be aware that your need to help can sometimes overrule the child and deny their right to have a 'say' over what is right for them. It may be better to wait for another opportunity and see if they are more receptive.

Sick children will have been through some rather unpleasant experiences. It is normal practice for blood to be taken from the heel of babies. Babies can develop an association of pain to anyone touching their feet. The feet / pain association can be lessened, or removed, once the child learns to link pleasure rather than pain via their feet. For some children, however, it is a step too far. It may take time and patience to overcome fears and concerns about their feet being touched. Children react to situations instinctively and their responses are not a planned or intentional reaction to you. Do not take it personally if they react badly. Take your time and have another go later.

Note:

Premature babies may either enjoy or dislike Reflexology treatments and so it is kind to just try a little (if practical) and see / notice how they respond. Premature babies are not only separated from their Mothers in order to receive vital care but also have a huge number of unpleasant procedures when compared to healthy babies who stay with their mothers. Some babies may experience Reflexology as calming and soothing, whilst others may experience it as one more intrusion they could do without.

Try it and see, as those who can accept it, really seem to enjoy it and benefit physically and emotionally.

Tip - Babies will show distress through their feet by pulling away their big toes.
Any dorsiflexion (pulling back) of the Hallux (big toe) should be noticed, registered and acted upon. Although it may be tempting to carry on as 'it will do them good' it is important for the future relationship between you and the child that you pay attention to their needs.

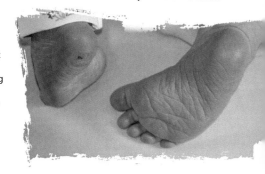

Assessment Process

Create an opportunity for communication with the child either via eye contact or the way that you speak. Keep your tone soft, reassuring and kind. Remember to move slowly in front of the face of a baby so that he / she can take their time to develop their focus. Rapid movements can be frightening for a baby. The way in which you conduct the assessment process can demonstrate your appreciation, sensitivity and care for the child. It is important to take your time when assessing a baby or child's feet as a rapid, perfunctory or rushed attitude can be very unsettling.

Ensure that you are paying attention to everything that can provide you with information including the child's life and environment. Notice the body language of both the child and the person(s) caring for them. Note their communication with each other, body contact and manner.

When assessing his / her feet, do this in a manner that does not feel invasive or scary, peering intently can be off putting! The 'scanning' of the child's feet can be done when you first see them i.e. in bed, walking or taking off his / her shoes and socks. Notice their toes, shape, colour and any distinguishing features. Pay attention to the fine details that can provide valuable clues to the inner workings, attitude and condition of the child. Make a visual assessment skilfully without it being too obvious. They could be worried about what you can see or what you have found.

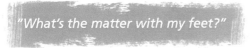

"What's the matter with my feet?"

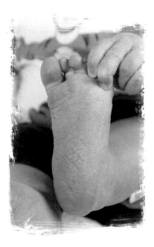

Notice:-

- Skin tone
- Texture
- Colour
- Markings
- Movements
- Reactions
- Temperature
- Skin condition

Keep a physical or mental note of this for later.

Ensure that your first touch is slow, gentle and is done with warm hands! This is when the child is assessing the quality of your touch and making decisions about whether they like it, if it feels safe and if they want more! You are also assessing the skin tone, texture and flexibility of their feet. This is all gleaned by noticing the subtle indicators revealed within their feet including the levels of flexibility or rigidity, moisture levels of the skin or the shape of the toes etc.

Initial Consultations

If you are treating someone else's child with Reflexology you need to be a fully qualified and fully insured practitioner. When treating babies or children it is essential to gather together all the available information on what the child's situation is, how they are and what is going on, before treating them.

Every case should be considered in its own right. It is essential that a full Initial Consultation is done for the child. All treatments must only be undertaken after a signed consent for treatment has been obtained from the parent / guardian. An initial consultation sheet should be used to obtain as much information as possible, in order to ascertain how best to treat the child. I find it helpful to say that the information I am requesting is 'so that I can work out how best to be able to treat your child.'

If the child is able to speak for themselves, then it is advisable to direct the questions specifically to the child, even if they can only answer just the briefest of questions (i.e. "what is your name?" / "do you know when your birthday is?". Very important questions are, "do you know why "X" has brought you here today?" or, "do you know what may happen while you are here today?" This gives you chance to find out what the child knows; what sense they have made of the information that they have been given or if they know anything about why they are here! They may have been playing or concentrating on something else when they were told about coming to see you. Therefore, having no idea why he / she is there or what may happen. Whatever he / she says provides you with a starting point to build a rapport and to communicate simply and directly with the child and to build a relationship with him / her. I like to think that it is possible, in many cases, to join forces with the child to help them with what they perceive they need. This may differ from why the parent / carer brought them to see you.

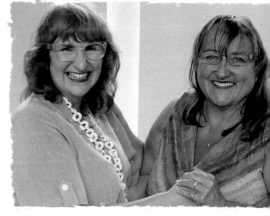

Example

My young client, Alex (7), was brought to see me by his mother. She had booked him in for a treatment as his knees were causing him pain and he had missed some days at school. When I asked him why he had come, he said that it was to make his feet better! I asked him if his feet needed to get better and he said "no - his feet were fine". So we clearly had a discrepancy here! Then I asked him if he thought there was anything we could do to make anything better. He said "no", so I asked him if he wanted to run better. He said "Yes" and I was able to follow on by saying; "so if Gentle Touch™ Reflexology could help you and your knees to work better, and help you to be able to run with your friends at school – would that be a good thing to try?" He said that he would like that. I then explained that the Reflexology meant that "I would be massaging his feet and that this special massage could send little helper messages to the bits that build his knees; help them to be stronger and help him to be better at running". When I asked him if he would like me to do this massage that is called Reflexology he grinned and said that he would.

During this consultation and discussion with Alex I kept the explanations simple whilst continuing to give him choices about what may or may not happen. My aim was for him to realise that we are working together as a team, in order to help him to be able to run faster and for longer. He really was not bothered about his knees (as his mother was) but he was interested in running better. He took the decision whether to proceed with the treatment thereby actively participating in the whole process.

In cases where the child is very ill, it may be that any communication would either be too tiring, inappropriate or just not possible.

 With young babies the responsibility lies with the parent, or carer, to provide the information. Any information that you require, that the child is not able to provide should be sought from the responsible adults caring for the child.

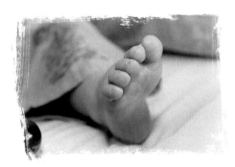

Who Benefits From the Initial Consultation Process?

If you are a Reflexologist it is essential that you gain the background and current information about your client. The initial consultation process allows the practitioner of Reflexology to assess the needs of the client and to begin the 'detective' process. This is where you can be pondering 'what is going on and why?' It is also the time when the baby / child and their parent/carer starts to form an opinion of you, your skills, professionalism and ability to help their child. This is a two way assessment process and both parties use this platform to create the relationship that follows. If this process is rushed, impersonal, too rigid in format or glossed over, then this can have a really detrimental effect on the future relationship between the client and the practitioner. Studies have shown that you only have a few seconds to make an impression. If these vital seconds are handled with lack of care then the client may decide that you do not know your subject or that you do not care. 'A good bedside manner is worth its weight in gold'. It can be hard to change someone's opinion, so it is worth investing extra time and energy at the beginning to set the rest of the treatment process off to a good start.

Aim to keep the consultation specifically relevant to them and not just filling in a pre-printed sheet. If you are a Reflexologist who uses a standard sheet then I suggest that you ensure that the form fits the client, and not the other way round with the client fitting the form!

A competent, personalised and appropriate initial consultation process can be the beginning of making a real difference. It is the foundation of healthy practice.

What Type of Information Should Be Requested in the Initial Consultation?

The basic information that you require includes the child's name, address and date of birth. I also recommend asking for two contact telephone numbers in case you need to get hold of them at short notice. It is now much more common practice to ask for email addresses too (remember to comply with any data protection legislation that relates to you).

It is a good idea to start with a 'general question' that can open up the whole proceedings. Something like, "what are you hoping to gain today by coming for this treatment of reflexology?" This will give you a place to start your 'detective' work and where you can start to create the plan (in your head) of what type of treatment you will conduct; what factors may be implicated here and what advice you may be offering in the future.

This is also a time when you find out about the client's expectations too. A parent may be thinking that there is nothing that reflexology can do and yet you know (perhaps from previous experience of the same or similar) that this may not be the case. Alternatively, it can be that they are praying that you will 'cure' a very sick child.
It is helpful to know roughly what they may be thinking, hoping for, or if they have any misconceptions about Reflexology. It gives you the chance to allay any fears and to be open and honest about the potential and scope of the treatment.

The answer to your initial question will start to set the scene and gives you an opportunity to discuss the case more openly with the clients, as you already have an idea of where they are coming from in terms of their expectations. Managing people's expectations is very much part of the role of a Reflexologist and this should be thoughtfully and sensitively handled. Always keep their reason for coming uppermost in your mind and tailor the treatment and advice specifically to their case.

Always ensure that you find out about any conditions, illnesses and accidents etc that the child may have had in the past, as well as any conditions occuring. It is helpful to note which side of the body they relate to. The Initial Consultation will provide valuable information about what is happening regarding their home circumstances, their general health, and their medical condition. It can also provide an insight into what might be happening emotionally and energetically.

When asking about the child's health; it helps to know

- What medication they are taking
- What treatments they are having (or are scheduled to have)
- Does anyone else in the family have anything the same or similar?
- Has anyone in the past had the same issues?

The Initial Consultation discussion may highlight certain conditions and links that can provide a clue as to what is going on. It can be very stimulating to start to put the pieces of the puzzle together, and to be able to work out what the issue may be about, as well as finding creative ways to solve it (or at least assist you to gain an insight into what may be the root cause). See pages 117 – 119 for more information.

Example - Shoulder Pain

My client Emma (12) arrived quite breathless for her treatment. She was highly apologetic that she was late as she had come straight from school. I had not appreciated that she would be coming alone and had assumed that she would be accompanied. She explained that it has been necessary to pop home on her way to see me to give her Mother some tea. Emma and I chatted for some time and it soon became clear that she is a very capable young girl who manages a huge amount of challenges in her life. Her Mother is disabled and she pops home at lunchtime to give her Mother lunch and then does the dinner when she gets in from school. Her Aunt had made the gift of the treatment as Emma had fallen and hurt her right shoulder and this was causing her pain. During our brief discussion Emma and I decided that it would be better for her to come again another day, when she had more time and when her Aunt could come and support her. This is a clear example of how someone's circumstances relate to their condition. Shoulder problems relate to 'having the world on their shoulders' and her right shoulder relates to having too much to do. So the fact that she had pain in her shoulder relates to the pain of her having so much responsibility.

Also see DVD – Success Tips for Reflexologists for another example

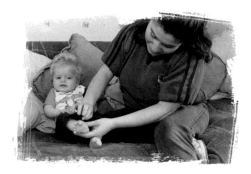

Mother / Mother Figure Connection

It helps to pay attention to what is being experienced by the child and see how it may possibly relate to the mother. There is a school of thought that suggests that if the mother is struggling in some way, then the child may subconsciously manifest something as well. It can be seen as both getting the same (or similar) condition, or both having health challenges at the same time. I remember when one of my sons was injured and I wanted to think it was just an accident

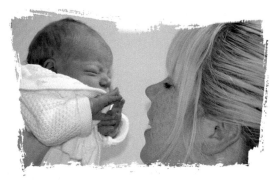

(which it was), but I also realised that I was hurting about something too. Now both of us were hurting – so that was possibly fair in a child's eyes. It is a controversial thought, but one that you may, or may not, find useful. It is worth noting if there is potentially something relating to treating the child that is also supportive of the mother / mother figure. A loving intention to be there for all concerned is one reason why both parties may sometimes opt for treatment. On a number of occasions I have found that once the child is gaining benefit from the treatment then the mother may also see the potential for herself too. If a child is ill or struggling then it is very stressful for the relatives as well. Being able to use the same or similar treatments to support everyone is a wonderful way to help both the child and their whole family.

There are many potential layers of possible causes, implications and meanings to consider. It can make the detective work all the more interesting as you begin to recognise the various reasons why something may, or may not be a contributing factor. Therefore finding it simpler to see through to the real issues. Once the deeper issues are recognised then it is easier to tailor your treatment, advice and care for your client, (see more information on links on pages 117 – 119).

Sixth Sense

I find it very helpful to ask the parent / carer what they think is the cause or trigger etc for the child's condition. It may be surprising how often the parent has an idea of what may be related. They may have dismissed the idea but actually be right in their assumption or intuition. If you do not ask, then you miss an invaluable source of information.

Parental Consent

If you are a Reflexologist and treating someone else's child, always ensure that you obtain signed parental consent or, if the child is in hospital, you must gain the relevant consultant's permission before treating.

Example of a Parental Consent Form:

Treatment Consent Form

I _____

Give consent for _____ (Practitioner)

To treat my child _____ with Reflexology

I acknowledge that this treatment is not a replacement for any orthodox or prescribed medical treatment and advice. I undertake to take full responsibility for giving the above named child access to medical care and attention. I will notify the above named practitioner if there are any changes to the details provided during this initial consultation. I acknowledge that there are no guaranteed outcomes and that I take the responsibility for requesting this treatment for the above named child. Reflexology is a complement to medical help and not a replacement for it. (If you are in any doubt please seek appropriate medical advice).

Relief from Eczema

"My Son has eczema and we feel that Reflexology has made a really big difference to him. It hasn't just treated his symptoms, it's also treated him."

Mother J

Responses and Reactions

Babies and children will often respond in a more obvious manner than adults to treatments. This means that a child might become very excitable or withdrawn and quiet following a treatment. These are normal responses. The child, however, may be exhibiting a different response from what is usual for them and this may cause the responsible adult concern. A child's response is likely to be pure, instantaneous and therefore gives us honest feedback!

Always ensure that you discuss possible responses and reactions to the treatment with the adult carer in order to allay any concerns. They may need to call you to discuss their child's behaviour or reaction following the treatment.

Take time for anyone to ask questions before the treatment begins and after the conclusion of the treatment.

Treating the reflex points outlined in the treatment routine is dependent on you being able to reach / follow where the child's foot is. They have a delightful tendency to have dancing feet! One minute their feet can be in front of you, and the next they have moved and their feet are up and out of reach! Obviously it will also depend on how well or tired the child is as to how much their feet wriggle about.

Do whichever reflexes you can manage whilst keeping a good rapport with the child. If necessary reduce, pause or close the treatment until the child re-engages with the process later on. In some cases the child needs to show their independence. The more you allow them to have their freedom, the more likely it is that they will then allow you the space and positioning in order for you to continue with the treatment. A child may need extra time to gain their confidence in you and trust the fact that this treatment does not hurt and can make them feel good.

Be aware that parents / responsible adults will sometimes try to discipline / restrain the child whilst thinking they are helping you. They may grip the child's legs or feet and try to keep them still. It is therefore useful to state at the beginning of the consultation that free movement of their child's feet is perfectly acceptable.

Duration and Frequency of Treatments

The length of time that it can take to do a treatment for a child will depend on it's age, health and the size of their feet / hands.

A child that is very sick may need less treatment (but more frequently) than a healthy and energetic child.

A very young baby	A full treatment on a tiny baby's feet will take 5 - 10 minutes
3 - 9 months	A full treatment will take approximately 10 - 15 minutes
9 - 12 months	A full treatment will take approximately 15 - 20 minutes
12 - 18 months	A full treatment will take approximately 20 - 25 minutes
18 months - 3 years	A full treatment will take approximately 25 - 30 minutes
4 - 10 years	A full treatment will take approximately 30 - 45 minutes
10 - 16 years	A full treatment will take approximately 45 - 60 minutes

A very sick baby or child must have the care of the appropriate medical professionals, however they may also benefit from shorter but more frequent treatments (2 - 3 minutes), two or three times a day.

It may take 45 minutes to do 20 minutes of effective treatment for a 3 year old. Aim to leave time to settle the child, to explain and to pause as necessary. If you work at their pace, the results can be much better as you get the chance to build a better rapport. The trust built can allow you to conduct more treatments and for longer, so it is a wise investment of time to take it at their pace.

"My son was dreadfully affected by Eczema when we first took him for Reflexology. His skin was in a dreadful state. The Reflexology treatments and advice that we received have transformed him. His skin is now absolutely fine and he hardly ever has any flare-ups now."

Mother B

Reflexology can be part of a treatment or become part of their everyday routines. It can be done when the child is getting ready for bed, relaxing at home, preparing for the day or a special event. One of my clients uses it as a treat for special occasions. Another client always books her children in for treatments before any school tests or examinations as their 'luxury' so that they are cool, calm and collected before they start.

When parents wish to know more and learn a few simple moves / techniques it can be rewarding and connecting for both parent and child. Watching a child struggle is painful and hard but easier if the parent can at least do, or offer, something that can help.

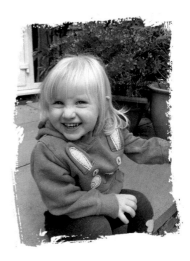

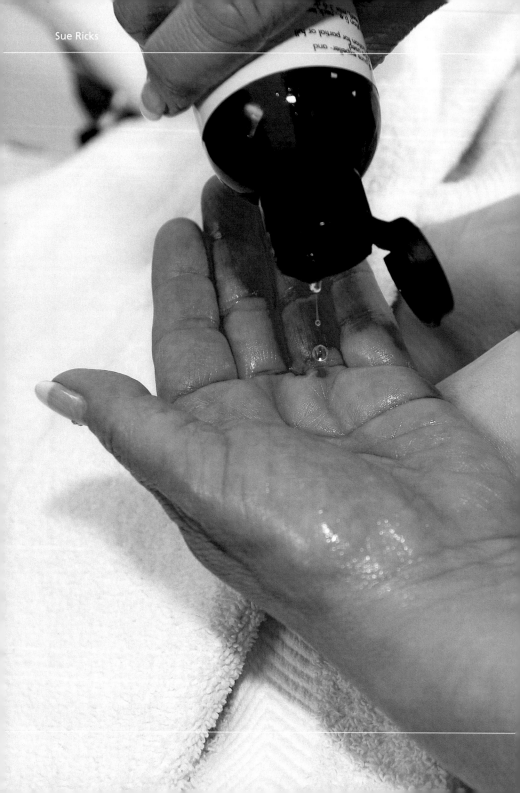

Getting Started

This is a recommended Gentle Touch™ Reflexology treatment practice for use when working with babies and children.

Creating the Best Environment

Take time to make the area where you do your treatments the most comfortable, relaxing and nurturing area possible. This benefits both you and the child.

Also remember that your role in Reflexology is to act as a facilitator for the child / client's own healing. Their healing response comes from within.

If you are treating at home or in some other location you will need to gather together the items that you will be using.

Baby

- A hand towel for under their feet and another towel for you to use
- Oil or lotion
- Small, safe & clean toys (as appropriate)

Child

- Pillow for under their head
- Second pillow for under their feet (if necessary)
- Hand towel for under their feet
- One as a 'modesty' towel to put over their legs
- Third towel for you to use
- Oil / lotion - see checklist to ensure contents are non toxic
- Safe and hygienic games, toys, books (as appropriate)

You can treat in a variety of locations from everyday places such as the sofa or the bed, or taking a child to see a professional practitioner who is experienced in treating children.

Your role in Reflexology is to act as a facilitator

A Reflexology practitioner might be able to set up their work space to be ready for all eventualities. The seating arrangements can be easily accommodated for various ages of children attending the clinic (or for home visits).

 A variety of options include:

- A good quality Reflexology chair
- A recliner chair
- A massage couch
- A Reflexology stool

I recommend a number of chairs / recliners including the La Fuma or Wellbourn chair. When you use a recliner chair it enables you to be at a similar height to the child or adult holding the child. It is a very comfortable position for the client and is easy and safe for them to get on and off. I recognise that many Reflexologists use massage couches. I, however, prefer proper recliner chairs – it is a personal preference.

Pillows

When using a pillow behind a child's head, ensure that it is the appropriate thickness as some pillows are too thick to use behind the neck of a young child. The best guide is to notice the angle of the child's head and the position of their neck when the pillow is behind their head. If their head is leaning forward then the pillow required needs to be thinner. I find it helpful to have three different thicknesses of pillows ready for my client's various needs.

When you have checked that you have everything to hand and are ready to start treating the child, begin by wrapping the child's feet slowly and gently. If it is too rushed it can be intimidating.

Coping with Exams

"My daughter had been panicking about taking her exams. My friend recommended Reflexology and it has surprised me how much it has helped."

Father S

Towels

The towels can be placed under their feet and then wrapped around them in a 'three part fold' before you start and when you finish treating. This 'three part fold' keeps the towel in position and yet their feet are not 'bound'. It looks a smartly folded towel and keeps a sense of protection for the child. When you open the towels; only open just enough to treat (unless their feet open it for you). There is a greater sense of protection when anyone's feet remain partially covered. The child might feel vulnerable if the towels are completely opened out.

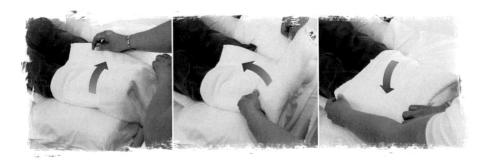

Size of Feet

The size of a baby or child's foot makes a difference as to how you treat. Quite simply, the older a child, the larger their foot and so the clearer the reflex points are to locate. A small movement and touch with your thumb on a tiny baby will cover a large percentage of the child's foot and, therefore, relate to several reflex areas of the body at once.

Work as many areas as you are able to, according to the child's attention, the size of your fingers and the size of their feet. It does not matter if you have small or large fingers either. Some of the most beautiful baby treatments that I have witnessed have been done by both delicate fingers but also by huge chunky male hands! One of my graduates works putting lead onto old English country houses and also works the magic of Gentle Touch™ Reflexology on tiny tots too. He has large dependable fingers that can work little miracles.

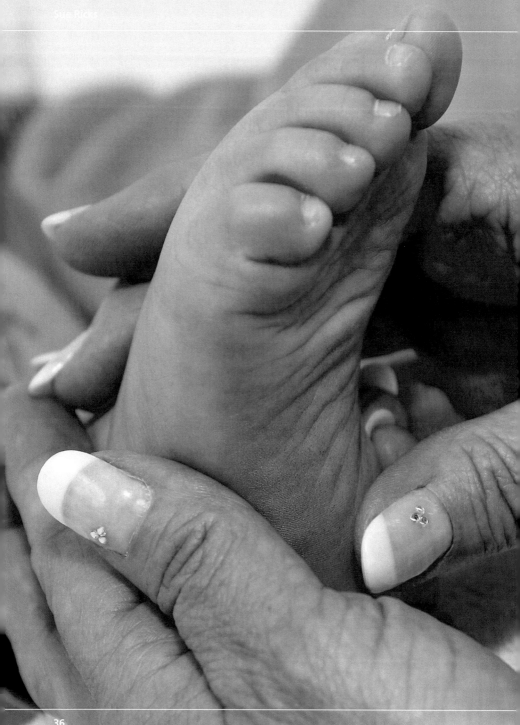

The Treatment

First Touch of a Baby or Child's Feet

The element of touch is so essential and once the first contact has been made with the child's feet you should endeavour to maintain some level of contact with their feet until the treatment has been completed.

The start of the treatment could be thought of as 'just a start of doing a treatment'. It is actually a very significant moment that could be easily missed. It is the moment at which the child first gets a chance to assess you and how you care for them. You are also assessing them. Vital clues as to how they are coping and responding are revealed. Take a short while to pay attention to this first contact as you never get this moment again.

Relief from Stomach Ache

"My daughter began experiencing some very unpleasant stomach aches when she was twelve. We always seemed to be either at the doctors or the hospital but no one could tell us what was wrong or was causing them. I wish I had known about reflexology before as after only the first treatment she felt better. We hardly ever get problems now but if we do get another bad spell this is quickly resolved by a treatment."

Mother A

Contra Indications – (when you should not treat)

Reflexology is not (and cannot be used as) an alternative to orthodox medical treatment and advice. If your baby or child is unwell, you should seek professional medical advice and care. It is important that you do not treat if there is an indication of high fever, thrombosis or a blood clot. If in any doubt consult an expert.

Beginning the Treatment

When you are ready to start the treatment, put sufficient oil on your hands to lubricate them freely. Calmly and gently unwrap the child's feet. Place your hands on the top of their feet, rest your hands there for a few moments, and then slowly move your hands down toward their ankles and away from their toes (i.e. from below the toes towards the ankle and leg). Some children will be worried that you will tickle their toes. By moving away from the toes you allow them to settle down and get used to your touch. Additionally, they will begin to relax into the treatment and you can start to assess their feet.

Sweep your hands down and around the ankles. Make sure that your hands are well-oiled and proceed to smooth oil over the top of the foot only. You may need to re-oil your hands once you have made these initial moves. You can maintain physical contact with them by keeping one hand on their foot and turn it palm up to receive the oil that is poured into a cup shaped hand.

It is important that you remember to keep paying attention to the child and maintain regular eye contact. A few reassuring smiles go a long way! You can tell a great deal by keeping eye contact. The eyes are known as the 'windows of the soul' and will give you valuable feedback about how they are feeling and responding to the treatment.

Tip - Ensure that you look at them before speaking as they may have fallen asleep since you last looked! If they have their eyes closed remember any questions that you might have until the completion of the treatment i.e. after their rest time. It is also possible that they might have their eyes open, but have a glazed expression as if day dreaming. This is a great sign of relaxation so do not disturb them by speaking (unless absolutely necessary).

When you touch a reflex point, i.e. a specific place on the foot, you are actually working with that part of their body. A good way of thinking is, 'Peter's head', rather than 'the big toe', as the big toe (Hallux) is the reflex area relating to Peter's head.

Go with the Flow

One of the best things about Gentle Touch™ Reflexology is that this routine is a very flowing set of techniques that gives you the chance to let the treatment just flow. It is more about the flow and encouraging the child's spirit and energy to flow, rather than the practicalities of getting it 'just right'. Obviously doing it 'right' is important, but should not be focussed on, to the detriment of the flow. Sometimes people can be so concerned about getting it right that they either do nothing at all, or are so fixed in their heads that they lose the capacity to really feel and sense the treatment. This sensitivity is what Gentle Touch™ Reflexology is about. With practice this is how you will develop your senses to know how to touch, where to touch, what pressure to use, or even not to touch (and do aura work instead) and so much more. The flowing nature of the treatment is the best thing to aim for. If in doubt about where to touch, or what comes next, just keep your hands and fingers moving in lovely massaging strokes over the foot until you reconnect with what comes next, or where you are working.

Stay as relaxed as possible and allow the treatment to flow. Once it is flowing you might find that you instinctively know more about where to go and what to do. Sometimes your head might be your own worst enemy as you try to do it 'right'. Do your best to work at a relaxed pace as too rapid an approach may cause the child to feel unsettled or 'wound up'!

Whole foot / hand = whole body = whole person / baby / child

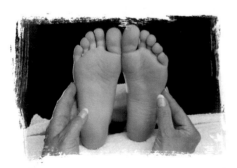

"I'm really glad I had my treatments as I don't get my headaches any more."

Sam, aged 10

What to Feel

When you are touching the baby or child's foot / hand, there are a multitude of different things to feel for in Gentle Touch™ Reflexology. Some are obvious whilst some are quite subtle.

The subtle indications are quite difficult to describe due the nature of their slight variations. Once you have had the chance to feel a few different babies or children's feet, or are used to your own child's feet you might start to notice the subtle changes and variations.

> Ideally the feet will feel smooth, warm and toned

If the area feels soft and also a little squelchy (as if there is a jelly-like pad in the skin) this is an indication of a potentially vulnerable area (a weak spot) that when taken care of, might settle down and not trouble the child, i.e. a latent condition.

If it feels soft and squelchy and is also a tiny bit more 'flushed' (pinker / coloured), then this may be an indication of inflammation that may be troubling the child i.e. it is an active condition.

If it feels 'empty', as if someone needs to pump it up a little (inflate), then this is an indication that the child's energy is low in this area. This may be because of an illness or maybe they 'used it up' as in:

- A youngster who is working hard to prepare for school examinations might have low energy over the crown of their head as they have used up all their 'thinking' energy.
- A child who is anxious or nervous over something then the energy of the solar plexus may have been "used up".

Some reflex areas of the skeletal system can feel sharp or jagged if there is a current challenge in a particular joint. In an older child or teenager you may feel that an area feels like smooth stone. This is often when their body has gone as far as it can with its healing of a particular area and thus 'sealed it over', leaving it feeling smooth and 'encased'. If you feel this then it relates to a condition, accident or injury from some time past.

After Treatment

Stages of Progress

It is normal for everyone to want an instantaneous result after a single treatment. However, it can take time. What many people initially miss is progress being made. Ideally we want three phases of progression.

1 Halt the decline
2 Keep this level (without the decline recommencing again)
3 An improvement

It is common for both clients and practitioners to fail to recognise Stages One and Two being achieved. Stages One and Two require a great deal of energy to obtain and should be acknowledged. When they are recognised this can give rise to more confidence that Stage Three, the desired outcome, might also be reached as well.

Sometimes it is the subtle benefits that can be missed, but these might be the most significant and important.

Right Hand Side vs Left Hand Side

The right hand or foot relates to the right hand side of the body and the left hand or foot relates to the left hand side of the body.

There is also a link to the type of issues that can specifically relate to one side of the body.

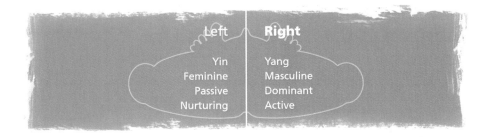

Left	Right
Yin	Yang
Feminine	Masculine
Passive	Dominant
Nurturing	Active

Descriptive Reference

Although I have endeavoured to use language that is simple and easy to understand I have, in some instances, used the following terminology to accurately identify the locations of certain reflex points.

- Plantar – sole of the foot / palm of hand
- Dorsal – top of the foot / hand
- Medial – inside of the foot (down from big toe / thumb to heel of foot / hand)
- Lateral – outside of foot / hand (from little toe / finger to heel of foot / hand)

Gentle Touch™ Reflexology Treatment Routine for Babies and Children

This is a full routine that follows the treatment through all reflex points.
The treatment flows from one foot to the other and back again. This continuous flow from area to area takes you through a full treatment routine. If you only have a short amount of time you can do a shorter treatment as outlined below.

- Head
- Solar Plexus - Page 53
- Spine - Page 59
- Pelvis (Hold) - Page 75
- Bowel (Sweep) - Page 78

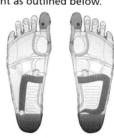

Head (including the pituitary)

The reflex points for the head and neck are found on;

- The big toes (Hallux) on both feet
- The thumbs on both hands
- The right foot / hand has reflex points that relate to the right hand side of the head
- The left foot / hand has the reflex points that relate to the left hand side of the head
- All areas of the head and brain have reflex points situated in the big toe / thumb therefore it is useful to work as many areas of the big toe / thumb as possible
- The base of the big toe / thumb represents the neck area

The top of the big toe / thumb has the reflex points for the top of the head (cerebrum) moving down to the base of the big toe / thumb, which contains the reflex points for the lower part of the brain stem (cerebellum) and the neck. The occipital region is on the dorsal aspect just above the neck area (base of the Hallux / thumb).

The front (dorsal aspect) of the big toe / thumb has the reflex points for the front of the head and face. The nose is at the level of the nail bed, following down the front of the toe to the base of the toe / thumb, with reflex points for mandible, maxilla and mouth. The maxilla reflex is found at the top of the joint in the big toe / thumb, and the mandible reflex is found at the lower part of the big toe / thumb joint.

Start with the child's left foot (on your right). Work gently and slowly across the top of the big toe / thumb – their head / brain. *All techniques demonstrated on Babies & Children DVD 1. Available through suericks.com.*

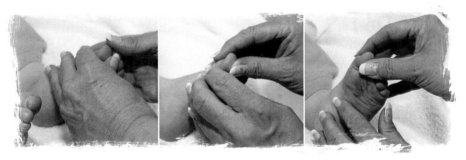

Slowly work across all of the head areas on the sole of the big toe (plantar aspect) and then work through to the area at the base of the big toe (neck). Gently touch the child's toe and gradually feel each area, moving in a line from left to right. Move down and work the next "line" until you have reached the base of the big toe. Then work (gradually feel down) the side of the toe using your fore or little finger. Only work between the toes if there is room.

HEAD

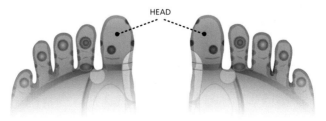

With small babies just work gently down the top to the bottom of the toe and as far as you can access.

Ages 8 onwards. A child changes through natural cycles of growth and development at different ages dependant on gender. This hormonal development can become noticeable at different ages and also be different in other cultures too. The levels of hormonal (endocrine) activity will vary from child to child. It is also frequently earlier in girls than in boys and so the reflex points will show different levels of activity.

Pituitary – The reason why we pay so much attention to this reflex area is because the pituitary is where all the hormones, that do so much to keep us healthy, are produced, and released. It affects just about everything in a growing child.

Pituitary and Hypothalamus. These are so close together that it is not possible to distinguish them separately, (therefore it is just the pituitary that is mentioned). The pituitary is found in the slight indentation on the side of the big toe just above the joint. The second location of the pituitary is in the centre of the swirls at the centre of the print of the hallux. If the pituitary reflexes are enlarged, prominent, pink in colour or harder to the touch, then it is an indication that the Endocrine system is out of balance. During periods of intense hormonal activity, i.e. the onset of puberty, the menses (periods) may also feel 'fizzy' or 'active' as well as pink and pronounced. If it feels 'empty', then this is an indication that it is not functioning to its peak potential. A little gentle stimulation might be required.

The big toe / thumb also represents the whole body in 'miniature'. This is why some children feel the effects of the treatment in areas other than the head at the commencement of the treatment.

If you only have a couple of minutes available to treat a baby or child it is helpful to treat the big toes / thumbs, followed by solar plexus (see page 122). This will provide an effective treatment for the whole baby, or child, if a full treatment is not possible.

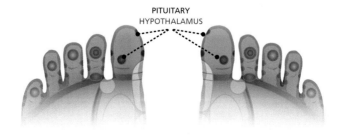

PITUITARY
HYPOTHALAMUS

Temporomandibular Joint (TMJ)

The TMJ is the joint between the temporal region of the skull and the mandible – otherwise called the jaw. It is an area commonly associated with stress 'grit your teeth and get on with it.' It's also an area of tremendous growth and activity in a child, as their milk teeth and then adult teeth are growing. Lots of energy is needed for this. Tooth ache is very common – see page 87.

The reflex point for the Temporomandibular Joint (T.M.J). is half way down the sides of the big toe / thumb, at the level of the toe / thumb joint. It is a very important area, as it is through the mouth of a baby or young child that they begin to build a picture of the world and gain information about their surroundings. Both babies and young children put just about everything into their mouths to check it out!

Older children may have become tense and have developed tension in the TMJ. If you place your index fingers either side of the TMJ and then gently hold the joint, whilst using a light rolling action, this can be relaxing and soothing for the child. This is also a good technique for use on airplanes (or in lifts) when the pressure changes. You can also do the same movement on the thumb. Locate the joint of the thumb and gently hold the area between your two index fingers or thumb and index finger on one hand, move your fingers in a rolling (round and round) action.

 If this joint is marginally displaced it can have a radical effect on the individual's well-being. There are thousands of nerve endings passing through this joint (it is known as the principal receptor area). It is important that the TMJ is noted because, if it is out of balance, the energy throughout the individual may be affected and every other area of the skeletal system could also be out of balance.

The TMJ represents both energetic and skeletal balance.

If it feels rigid the child may be gritting their teeth physically, but also remember the phrase - *'grit your teeth and get on with it!'*

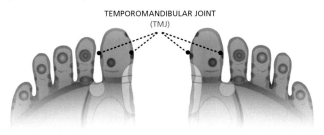

TEMPOROMANDIBULAR JOINT
(TMJ)

Neck

🖐 The reflex points for the neck are situated at the bottom of the big toe

Work round the base of the big toe using a circular massage movement. In very small children it will only be possible to do the tiniest of massaging movements here. However, this tiny amount of touch will be sufficient. Little massaging strokes all around the base of the big toe will be effective in working the reflex points for the neck area.

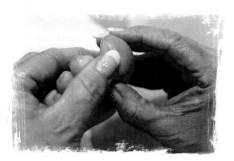

 Working across the base of the Hallux also takes in the cerebellum, all the neck areas and brainstem. Gently separate the big toe from the other toes and work down between the big toe and first small toe. Move to the outer side of the big toe to work down, taking in the reflexes for the side of the head and the start of the central nervous system. Move to the front of the big toe and work across the base of the nail progressing down towards the bottom of the toe. This can be done with one, two or three fingers together moving in a ripple walk across the toe. Take note of the maxilla (upper jaw) and mandible (lower jaw). This will show if there is a problem with the teeth.

Repeat Head and Neck on their Right Foot / Hand

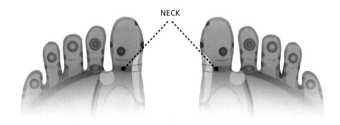

NECK

Small Toes

🖌 The small toes represent the sinuses, teeth and head region, also see location for the reflex points for the eyes, ears and Eustachian tubes.

🖌 Begin with the toes on the child's' left foot (on your right). Systematically work each toe in turn from the first toe to the little toe on the same foot. On each toe work the pad (sinus) of the toe down to the base of the toe.

🖌 Babies – run your fingers down the toes to the base of each toe (front and back). If the baby has a cold pay extra attention to the pads of the toes and do extra sinus drainage work downwards.

🖌 Toddlers and very small children – run your fingers down the toes from the tops of the toes to the base of the toe. Some young children have toes that 'spread out'. If so, work gently between the toes by lightly inserting your little finger in between the toes to work down the sides of the toes. Never force the toes apart. Only work if there is a natural space to work. If you have enough oil on your hands this becomes easier.

🖌 Older children – You can treat all four aspects (sides) of the toes more easily in older children, as the toes are longer and have more space between them. Notice how the toes fall and if any toe is pushed against the next, or if any one toe is especially rigid or curling. This is important and can reveal interesting information about foot reading – my next book 'Fantastic Feet' is all about foot reading and will be due out in 2010).

All four toes should be worked on the left foot before moving on to the right foot. The small toes can be worked faster than the big toes (but not too quickly).

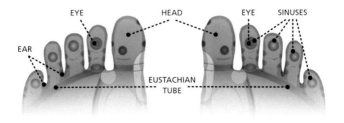

EYE   HEAD   EYE   SINUSES

EAR

EUSTACHIAN TUBE

Sinuses

🖐 The reflex points for the sinuses are located in the pads of each toe / finger

🖐 The reflex points for the sinuses behind the eye are on the first toe / finger

If there is any congestion in this reflex point it will contribute to pressure and discomfort around the eye. The sinus reflex points will feel soft, full and 'squidgy' if the child has a cold or inflammation of the sinuses. Thorough work of these reflex points will often relieve sinus symptoms during a treatment. Lots of gentle smoothing down the toes; especially massaging the pad of the toe, followed by further smoothing down, is a super way to help a child who is blocked up with a cold and struggling to breathe easily. It is possible for children to notice that they can breathe more easily during, or immediately after a treatment.

> If a client has repeated bouts of catarrh or colds it is worth considering if this might be because of a dairy intolerance or sensitivity (see page 92 for more information)

Eyes

There are a couple of reflex points that relate to the eyes.

🖐 The eye itself, i.e. the eye ball, is found at the bottom of the pad of the first toe / finger

🖐 The eye socket (orbital cavity) is found at the bottom of the first toe / finger; where the toe joins the foot

Ears

The reflex points for the ears are in more than one location. An ear is a complicated organ with many different areas and functions and the reflex point locations vary too.

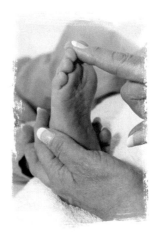

- The main areas for the ears are in between the third and fourth, and fourth and fifth (little) toes.

- The other location is at the actual location on the head i.e where the TMJ reflex points are located either side of the big toe / thumb, at the level of the joint.

The area in between the toes (either side of the fourth toe) will often feel 'gritty or knobbly' if there is a problem with their ear. If the child has had ear infections, is experiencing discomfort or is pulling at their ears, lightly hold the area at the base of the fourth toe (or finger). Hold steadily for about 30 - 60 seconds. Ideally hold and then follow with gentle massage to soothe and smooth the area. This helps the stagnated energy and reflex points to recommence a natural flow.

Also notice the area at the bottom of these toes where they join the foot. If they are 'lumpy' work the area and then run your thumb over to smooth. This will activate and then sedate the reflex area, thus encouraging a healing response.

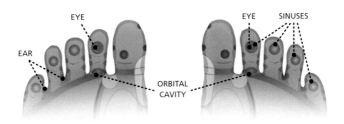

Eustachian Tubes

The Eustachian tubes are the fine tubes that connect your ears, nose and throat.

🖐 On the foot / hand it extends the whole way around the base of the little toe / finger and across and under the back of all the other toes / fingers.

Start at the bottom of the little toe and gently but sensitively move your thumb along under the toes in a similar way that a caterpillar moves along the ground. This is called a 'thumb walk'. Go as far as the gap between the big and first toe, BUT not into the gap (Thyroid reflex point). Ensure you work along the line immediately under the base of the small toes. Work along the line several times to ensure adequate drainage of the Eustachian tubes. Gently massage any areas of 'resistance' and return to them later in the treatment if necessary. Ensure that your thumb is tilted in towards the toes. This is in order to get into that essential area for effective drainage for the child.

Teeth

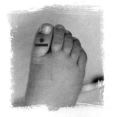

The reflex points for the teeth are found in two places:

🖐 Across the front of the big toe / thumb (across the top and bottom of the joint of the big toe) that represents the Maxilla and Mandible reflex points.

🖐 On the sides of each toe. The first toe / finger equates to the front teeth, while the little toe equates to the back teeth. The top row of teeth are found at the upper toe joints, whilst the bottom teeth are found at the lower toe joints.

Repeat all Small Toes on their Right Foot (On your left).

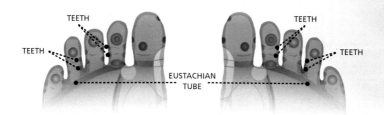

Lymphatic Drainage (Left and right foot)

The lymphatic system is complex. A simple overview is that it is the secondary circulatory system that is responsible for removing unwanted and unhealthy things from our bodies, i.e. cell waste and bacteria. The lymph nodes are like rubbish dumps, and the lymph vessels are like little roads leading to the rubbish dumps.

This technique is superb for eliminating waste products and assisting the body to cleanse itself.

There are two areas where we work the lymphatic systems:

* The upper / respiratory lymphatic system is across the top (dorsal aspect) of the foot, from just below the toes to midway down the foot.

* The lower / groin lymphatic areas are around the heel and ankle, then leading up to the mid section of the foot.

Upper / Respiratory Lymphatic Area

Place your thumbs horizontally (one above the other), under the ball of the foot (lungs). Your thumbs can then be used as a rest. Place your hands midway down either side of the foot. Gently sweep your hands up to the top of the foot, alternating one hand and then the other gliding up and across the top of the foot. These movements will allow you to gently separate the metatarsals as you massage, i.e. like a fan. Make this a beautiful flowing movement that both you and the child can enjoy!

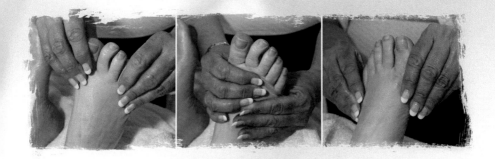

After approximately eight sweeps, start to drain up the gaps between the metatarsals (bones) / lymphatic channels, using right and / or left finger(s). Begin at the mid-line of the foot and work up towards the toes.

You can also do this on the hands by placing your thumbs under the palm of the hand and sweeping up the hand as described above.

It is helpful to do this sequence on the hands or feet slowly and sensitively.

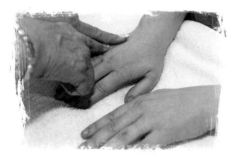

 Notice if there are any patches or areas of resistance. If any resistance is found this is an indication that there is a stagnation, or blockage, in the energy relating to the lymphatic system. Place your finger lightly on the affected spot. Wait for a short while and then see if the 'blockage' dissipates as this is often the case. If it is resistant to the single still touch, then repeat the lymphatic drainage sequence again and return to the area of imbalance.

Rest again.

If the area now clears, then the child may feel tingling throughout their body as the energy redistributes and balances itself. If the area of resistance remains, then it is likely the process will continue internally and that it will be clearer after a few days following the treatment. Make a note in your treatment records to assess the lymphatic system next time.

Solar Plexus (Relaxation Inducer)

The Solar Plexus is a ganglion of nerves at the bottom of the centre on your ribs – the place where you feel as if you have been 'thumped' when you are shocked. Working this area can really assist children to be calmer, more relaxed and contented. Sometimes people feel a warm glow when this area is eased.

- The reflex point for the solar plexus is in the centre of the foot or hand. In the little dip in the centre of the foot, (just under the ball of the foot).

- On the hand it is in the middle of the palm

With the feet facing you, place both of your thumbs, pointing up towards the top of the foot, in the resting place just underneath the line along the ball of the foot (See diaphragm line on chart). Hold this position until you feel that it is the right time to begin to gently ease into the solar plexus. Very gently 'press' / 'ease' into the area and notice when it feels right to stop. It is almost as if the child signals energetically when it is time to stop. Continue to hold for a short while and then either gently release, or ease a little further before releasing, whichever you sense is more appropriate. It is an extremely gentle but profound 'stress buster' button.

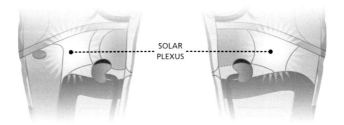

SOLAR PLEXUS

A child who is under a great deal of stress and strain may have a Solar Plexus which feels crunchy and crackly. Remember the phrase 'they are cracking up'!

Anyone who is feeling over whelmed and emotional or energetically exhausted may have a solar plexus that feels empty. When you place your thumbs on the area there will be no resistance / no barriers / nothing there.

Feel the 'texture' through a gentle rocking movement into the Solar Plexus. If it is very resistant repeat a gentle but penetrating slow rock into the Solar Plexus two or three times. Repeat this technique several times during the treatment if necessary.

Shoulder (Left foot)

 The reflex point for the shoulder is the area under the little toe / finger

The shoulder reflex is found all around the area under the small toe / little finger. Gently massage the whole joint on one foot / hand and then work both shoulder reflex points at the same time if appropriate. Any tension or rough areas that you feel here relate to some shoulder irregularity or strain with the child. This could be sign of either physical or emotional strain, i.e. taking the world on their shoulders and having to cope with a great deal.

The reflex point for the scapula (shoulder blade) is the triangular area under the little toe (planter). The clavicle runs just under the little and next toe (on the dorsal aspect). Roll your fingers around the left shoulder first. Assess how well aligned it is. Is it protruding, smooth or rough? If it is rough but puffy it is likely to be painful. Compare them with each other and check for symmetry.

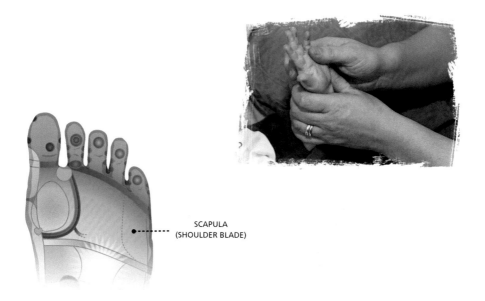

SCAPULA
(SHOULDER BLADE)

Arms / Elbow

The reflex points for the arm and elbow are down the outside (lateral) edge of the feet / hands.

* The arm starts just below the shoulder reflex and continues to the dip just above the joint of the fifth metatarsal. This is the bony area mid-way down the outside of the foot.

* The elbow reflex is in the dip / dent just above the joint of the fifth metatarsal.

Gently walk your fingers down the outside of the foot and into the dip above the joint of the fifth metatarsal. When you have 'felt' down the area you can follow it up with a series of massaging movements of small circles down the side of the foot / hand.

Continue with a gentle caterpillar movement feeling down the outside of the foot to the area just above the fifth metatarsal joint (elbow). Occasionally a strained shoulder joint or fracture can be felt as a 'cartilaginous feel' or knotty muscles in this area of the foot.

Hand

* The reflex point for the hand is on the dorsal aspect of the foot and is at right angles to the elbow reflex point. (As in the natural shape and angle of the arm with the elbow bent.)

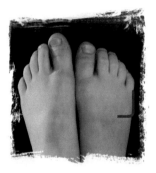

If the child has damaged their hand then it is good to work the corresponding reflex points, the reflex points for the hand can be found on the foot! Any area of soft tissue damage will be quite small and can be felt as a slightly puffy / 'squelchy' area. It might also be a tiny bit pink in colour too. Injuries affecting the bones can feel gritty, puffy or bony. It is often helpful to compare the reflex point for both hands together in order to feel the subtle differences between the two. It is frequently the subtlest of changes that indicate the precise location of the reflex points.

Knee

The reflex points for the knee are found in two locations:

- One area is at the level of the fifth metatarsal- all around the joint

- The second reflex area is along the Achilles tendon

    - The back of the knee joint is found on the back of the foot / hand (plantar aspect)
    - The patella (knee cap) is on the side of the foot / hand (lateral aspect)
    - The front of the knee is on the front of the foot / hand (dorsal aspect)

The knee is a surprisingly large area and takes up bit more room than might be expected. Working in smooth strokes and feeling around the whole knee area can often help to locate areas of tension, strain or lack of energy / power. This is an especially important area as the baby / child will be using their knees for crawling or walking. The growth plates are under great strain through to their teens and on into adulthood. The legs / knees and skeletal system in general do an amazing job in developing and growing as baby / child's body ages. Reflexology can be a superb support for the body of the baby / child. In some cases the knees can show if the strain is too much. It is quite common for children to get 'growing pains' or painful knees and Reflexology can help to ease discomfort.

When I started working with children I was surprised at how many children had painful knees. Many times it was not specific but nevertheless still very common and a real nuisance to the child concerned.

Life-related / emotional implications of knee problems is that knees relate to moving forward, and being able to cope with the shocks in our lives. Our knees help and enable us to move forward whilst being our shock absorbers. When a child's knees are uncomfortable, or have become painful, it can represent that they are finding it difficult to move forward in life, or are finding growing older uncomfortable. Sometimes the added pressure or responsibility, reduction in parent contact time, etc. can be tough. It may happen at a time of school changes, family issues or house moving. It may also be friendship groups altering or preparing for examinations. The more painful the knees are, the more that it represents the degree to which the child is finding it increasingly difficult or painful. They may be hiding the issue, even from themselves, as they may be feeling that they have to cope. In reality they are finding the process of moving on, or forward, quite difficult. Consequently, it is wonderful if an adult is able to recognise the signs that the child's body is providing so that it can be addressed. Remember that the child may not be consciously aware of this. It may be that their body is alerting them to some worry that is subconscious i.e. behind the scenes. Painful knees are an important indicator of all the aforementioned issues and an important signal to recognise.

Knee reflexes on the foot

Work all around and underneath the joint of the fifth metatarsal on the foot, as this is the reflex point / area for the knee. The whole joint is the main reflex point for the knee. Work / feel around the joint and then gently massage the whole knee reflex area. This is the whole section around the joint. Also include the reflex area for the back of the knee (under the joint of the fifth metatarsal). It is often useful to compare the state of both knees by checking the reflex points on both feet at the same time.
An additional referral area for the knee is found on either side of Achilles tendon. Work steadily all around this area to improve both knee and leg function.

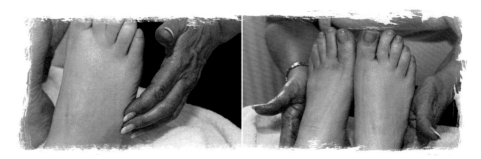

Knee reflexes on the hand

The reflex points for the knee are found mid way down the lateral aspect of the hand. Placing your finger or thumb half way down the outside of the hand is a good way of finding the knee reflex area.

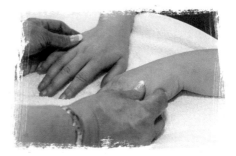

Leg / Hips / Pelvis

The reflex point for the leg / hips and pelvis are at the bottom of the outside edge (lateral) of the foot / hand.

🐾 The reflex points for the legs extend down from the knee reflex (the level of the fifth metatarsal joint mid way down the foot / hand) down to the bottom of the foot and round into the ankle / wrist

🐾 The secondary reflex areas are along the Achilles tendon at the base of the foot

Gently 'walk' your fingers along the outside edge of the foot from mid-way (knee reflex level), down to the bottom of the foot and around underneath the foot. Follow this with a massaging action and then little circles to the bottom of the foot. Finish with working all of the triangular area at the bottom of the heel and up to the ankle bone. Continue 'finger feeling' down the outside of the foot in a straight line, from the joint of the fifth metatarsal to the bottom of the heel area. The reflex points for the leg and hip continue down this line.

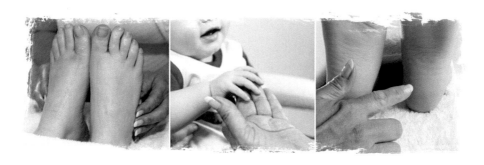

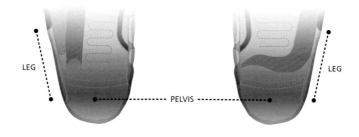

The hip is located in a curve under the ankle bone / wrist.

Again, work in a line to the bottom of the foot and then gently work the triangle between the ankle bone / wrist and the bottom of the foot / hand. This contains the reflex point for the pelvic region. Areas of pain and inflammation will feel hot and / or puffy. Other reflex areas for the leg extend further up onto the leg / wrist.

SPINE STARTS ------●

Spine

The reflex area for the spine is along the side of the foot / hand (medial aspect). It starts at the level of the TMJ (mid-way down the big toe / thumb) and continues all the way down to just above the bottom of the foot / heel area.

When holding the foot or hand, remember to check the level of pressure that you are using with your supporting hand and keep it light. You can hold without gripping as the hand or foot is not going to go anywhere – it is attached! A light and gentle hold gives the child a feeling of support and protection rather than being held in place. When you hold the foot / hand gently, it can then also represent being 'held'.

Hold the left foot / hand gently and positively and use two or three fingers to follow the line of the spine down the inside of the foot / hand. The spine follows the slightly bony ridge from just above the top of the base of the big toe / thumb to just before the bottom of the heel of the foot / hand. In a baby this feels much more soft and fleshy so just follow the same line down their tiny foot.

SPINE ENDS ------●

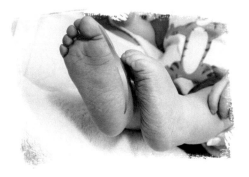

Using your fingers, walk down the spinal reflexes and feel for any irregularities. Work down the spinal reflexes two or three times. After each time, gently stroke upwards. Follow, if desired, with a three fingered vertical walk down the spine. This will allow you to note any irregularities. Any soft sockets or dish-shaped areas when associated with puffiness could be an indication of inflammation or vulnerable areas.

I have noticed that a surprising number of babies with sleep disturbances and who cry frequently have an enlarged and distinctly noticeable area on the reflexes for the lower spine (lumbar). The lumbar reflexes seem to be quite prominent and feel almost angular, with some extra associated puffiness. It is hard to describe, but when you have felt it you will know what it feels like! If the baby is unhappy, crying and does not like to be put down to sleep, give this technique a go. I have had so many superb results with it. I wonder if these new born babies actually have some kind of back trauma that is not obvious enough to be picked up conventionally after birth, but is uncomfortable or painful. Thus Reflexology treatment helps to assist them and encourages a healing response. Maybe if they have been in pain or discomfort the treatment can have a similarly rapid result that it does for some adults.

If you notice this prominent area, work your fingers slowly and steadily across and around it. Then lightly leave your finger on the area. If the baby / child seems to be sensitive to this level of touch, lighten your touch further. It is possible to have an effect, even if you are barely touching the foot. Close with the lightest and most loving touch / massage possible, to support both the baby and their struggling reflex areas.

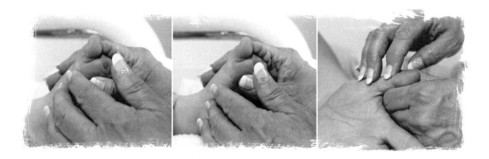

Follow the spine through its natural curvature encompassing the five regions:

- Cervical
- Thoracic
- Lumbar
- Sacral
- Coccyx

Feel for areas of irregularity, sensitivity, puffiness, lumps, bumps etc. Nodules, lumps and bumps often indicate injuries and disc damage. The older the injury the smoother they feel - more like stone, as if the body has sealed it over time. Aggressive or sharp ridges, bumps or lumps indicate current or recurrent back pain, possibly caused by injury or accidents. Areas of puffiness or redness show areas of inflammation. It is common to feel both enlarged and expanded reflexes with puffiness due to inflammation. Check for symmetry, alignment and texture. Irregularities need gentle and responsible attention as they may indicate anything from muscle weakness and strain to disc injuries.

Repeat the reflexes for the Spine on their Right Foot / Hand

"We often find that the diaphragm is not moving. The diaphragm is attached to the lower thoracic spine, and the front of the upper lumber vertebra which are also often involved."

"When this is rectified with extremely gentle, specific osteopathic treatment babies will usually become much more settled, with improvements in feeding and sleep pattern...."

"We also find that there may be insufficient flexibility in the base of the skull and the back of the head. This may be linked to a birth trauma, such as a particularly slow, or sometimes very rapid delivery, and can lead to them being an unsettled or colicky baby."

Nicholas Woodhead, Osteopath

Lungs (Left foot / hand)

🐾 The reflex points for the lungs are across the ball of the foot or fleshy part of the hand

There are some really lovely advantages that can be gained from working the lung reflexes. Not only are the lungs important physically, but also emotionally. Many children 'control' their breathing and hold their breath, or breathe quite shallowly, if they are anxious or stressed. Working along and over the lung reflexes can help a child's lungs physically and support them emotionally too. It can help them to be calmer and more relaxed.

Place your thumb or both thumbs on a larger foot, and move step by step down the ball of the foot to the line under the ball (or fleshy part of the hand). This reflects the diaphragm line.

Work down the lung reflex areas. Then use your thumb or thumbs to smooth up again. Begin at the lateral edge (shoulder reflex) and work across the ball of the foot by working down and then smoothing up. Continue to steadily work towards the medial aspect. Stop at the natural line / crease around the ball of the big toe joint.

'Smooth' the ball of the foot / hand. If the lungs are or have been affected by illness / infection, the reflex points will feel hard, crunchy or dense. The state of the lung reflex reflects the health, function and maturity of the lungs. Sometimes the lung reflexes show an irregularity in just one small location, or maybe just on one foot i.e. one lung only. Alternatively, it might be across the lung reflexes on both feet / hands i.e. both lungs are affected. The softer they feel the better condition the lungs are in. The lung reflex area may feel empty. This indicates that there is very low energy. A gentle or soothing massage may help to provide movement in energy, function and increase capacity for health. A child with asthma may have tight lung reflexes – see information on common conditions in the Conditions section on page 81.

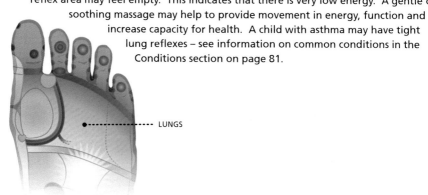

LUNGS

Thyroid

🖐 The reflex point for the thyroid is in between the big toe / thumb and the first toe / finger

The thyroid reflex point is part of the reflexes for the whole of the endocrine system. In Gentle Touch™ Reflexology it is located on the little pad between the big toe / thumb and the next toe / finger.

In babies and toddlers it is really tiny. There is no need to actively work this area as your fingers or thumbs will brush over it at some stage in a treatment. It is, however, an important reflex point for growth, as the thyroid releases growth stimulating hormone (GSH). A light and soothing slight massage of this area, followed by keeping your fingers still for a few moments, can be rebalancing for the thyroid reflex point.

In an older child, look at the reflex point. Is it regular in appearance, dipped or raised?

🖐 If it is uniform, smooth and regular in appearance; feels good with no bumps, lumps or irregularities, then the thyroid gland may be regarded as functioning well.

🖐 If the thyroid reflex area looks or feels dented, then the child's thyroid reflex may be over-active (hyper). If the thyroid reflex is dipped then gently rest your finger on the reflex point to calm and 'still' it.

🖐 If the thyroid reflex point looks, or feels, as if it is raised, then the thyroid reflex may be under active (hypo). If the thyroid reflex is raised then gently, but positively, massage the area between the big toe and the next toe. This increases the activity of the reflex point relating to the gland.

> Repeated treatments may be required

Each treatment may also indicate different stages and levels of activity, as the thyroid reflex point relates to a highly sensitive and energetically linked area. The thyroid is energetically linked to the throat chakra (an important energy centre), and is related to emotions around communication, including being able to communicate effectively and speaking out. (See more on Chakras on page 112)

Oesophagus / Trachea / Thymus

🐾 The reflex points for the oesophagus, trachea, thymus and para-thyroids are located in a line running down from the thyroid reflex point, around the ball of the big toe, to the medial aspect of the foot, i.e. around and underneath the ball of the hallux joint.

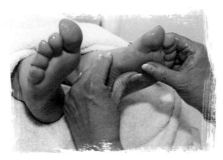

There is usually a natural crease indicating the location of this reflex area. The reflex starts at the top of the foot and flows towards the side of the foot, under the ball of the big toe. The trachea follows the same line and also branches towards the lungs (ball of the foot) at the bottom of the natural crease. Use your thumb to gently work down this natural crease line between the ball of the big toe and the ball of the foot. If the child has a throat related problem e.g. laryngitis, a sore throat, throat infection etc. these reflexes may feel swollen, lumpy, warm, knotty or grainy.

 Tracking down the line between zones one and two for the oesophagus and the trachea and you will also have worked the reflex point for the parathyroid.

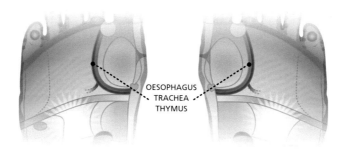

Heart

🐾 The reflex point for the heart is on the ball of the foot, under the big toe / thumb on both feet / hand. A key area of the child's heart reflex is at the bottom of the ball of the big toe / thumb.

Look at the reflex point and note any colour distortion or variations. Is the area raised, puckered, shiny, hot, blue, red or distinctly veined? If so, there may be some problems associated with their heart (unless it is caused by a shoe or sock!). Remember that emotions might also have an impact on their physical heart and the heart reflexes. When working the heart reflex area, always treat it with the respect that the child deserves. Always think "x's" heart (child's name), and imagine working on their physical heart. Work slowly, steadily and methodically over the entire heart reflex. Use both thumbs working with them placed side by side and gradually work down the area. Feel for any 'activity', movements, heat, lumps or bumps etc.

Peace Point (heart)

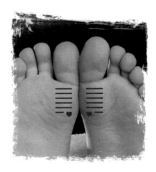

The peace point is a lovely delicate area that is at the bottom of the heart reflex.
'from the bottom of my heart'.

The heart is the centre of love and is fed by loving vibrations. Adults sometimes report a very subtle and 'nice' feeling when this point is lightly, lovingly and peacefully held. It is good to start young and offer the same loving support to young children too.

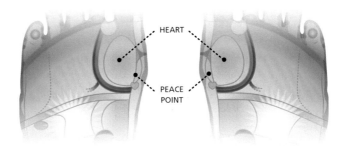

HEART

PEACE POINT

When you have finished working gently and softly over the heart reflexes, you may use the gorgeous peace point on the heart area. Very lightly place your thumbs on the bottom of the heart reflex. Think peaceful thoughts yourself and be 'still' inside. Hold this point for as long as you intuitively feel is appropriate. Observe any subtle changes in the child.

Note: only have your thumbs touching the feet while you do this linking technique.

Children and teenagers may have a line that cuts into the heart area and peace point if they have had a 'broken' heart. It is heart warming to watch this 'scar' heal over time. Soothe, caress and send love towards the person as you touch this area. A few lines mean they are very open-hearted and can get hurt easily. I have seen this line appear when any deep relationship breaks down or is lost e.g. break up of parents, finishing with a boy / girlfriend or loss of a pet.

Repeat lungs, thyroid, oesophagus, trachea, parathyroids, thymus and heart on left foot / hand

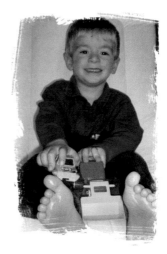

Liver

🐾 The reflex point for the liver is on the left hand side of the right foot / hand, just below or along the mid-line. It is triangular in shape, with the longest side down the side of the foot / hand (lateral edge).

The liver is obvious to see if it is enlarged, under pressure or is working hard. Place your thumbs side by side; gently work across and down the liver reflex area. Work across in lines, gradually working down the triangular shaped liver reflex area. In a tiny baby this is just one thumb touch as the reflex is so tiny.

Gall Bladder

🐾 This small duct is situated at the top of the liver reflex area. It is disc-shaped and sits along the mid-line close to the lung reflex area.

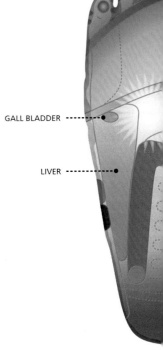

GALL BLADDER -----------●

LIVER -----------●

It is often visible if a child has recently had a particularly fatty meal or is sensitive to fats in their diet. Place your thumb on the gall bladder and work it normally.

Continue by working across the Solar Plexus reflex area (on the right foot / hand) using your thumbs.

A Calming Touch

"My twins love having their feet done. I have used it since they were about nine months old and immediately noticed a difference and we are still using it into their teens"

Mother D

Stomach (Right foot / hand)

The reflex point for the stomach is located on both the right and left feet / hands.

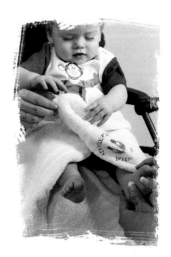

🐾 The lower half of the stomach (with the pyloric sphincter) is on the right foot / hand. The stomach reflex point is a dish-shaped area around, and underneath, the ball of the big toe / thumb joint.

Gently work this area checking for heat, grittiness, swelling, lumps or ridges. It can also feel empty or full. The stomach reflex point on a child who has just had a large meal will feel enlarged and 'active'. When treating a baby, simply touch and soothe the area with the tips of your thumbs.

Note: Children and parents / carers often refer to the whole of their digestive system as the stomach or tummy.

The reflex point for the duodenum is immediately to the left and below the stomach reflex.

Pancreas (Right)

The pancreas is also shown on both right and left feet / hands.

🐾 The reflex points for the tail of the pancreas are tucked in and under the stomach reflex points on the right foot.

Place your thumb under the stomach reflex point and gently roll up and under to locate the reflex point for the pancreas. It also extends out towards the solar plexus.

Move to Left Foot / Hand Reflex Points

Stomach (Left foot / hand)

Continue working across the stomach from the right foot.

* The left foot contains the reflex points for the top half of the stomach (with the cardiac sphincter)

  This reflex point links directly to the oesophagus

Work and then soothe this area. The stomach reflex point will feel bulky if the child has recently had a large meal. It will also feel bulky and lumpy if there is any kind of irregularity. Babies and children who experience feeding problems can be greatly helped by receiving Reflexology.

Pancreas (Left)

* The head of the pancreas shows on the left foot and is found just under the ball of the big toe.

The reflex point for the pancreas is found close to the medial edge, located mid-way down both feet. Work your thumbs gently round the area as shown on the chart.

Work across the Solar Plexus (on left foot / hand)

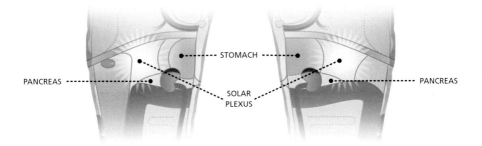

Spleen

- The reflex point for the spleen is a small irregular shaped area on the right hand side (lateral) of the left foot / hand

Work across the area with normal thumb presses. The spleen is usually spongy and soft. If it is working extra hard, i.e. to combat infection, then the Splenic reflex may feel warm, puffy and a little more pink than usual.

Move to the Right Foot / Hand Reflex Points

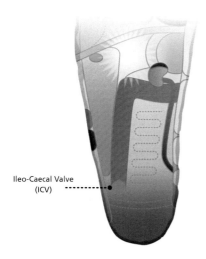

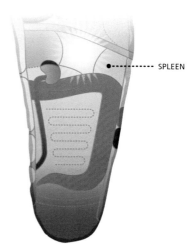

SPLEEN

Ileo-Caecal Valve
(ICV)

Ileo-Caecal Valve (ICV) / Appendix

This is the reflex point for the valve between the small intestine (ileum) and large bowel (caecum). It is important that the flow is uninterrupted and that the function of the valve is effective.

🦶 The reflex point for the I.C.V is felt as a small dish-shaped area two thirds of the way down the left hand edge (lateral aspect) of the right foot.

Place your thumb on the Ileo-caecal valve and gently press in and around the area. Many bowel problems, including flatulence (wind), colic and constipation, may be eased by working the I.C.V. and the rest of the bowel area.

 The ileo-caecal valve (I.C.V) can be an incredibly important point for Reflexologists. If there is any imbalance in the I.C.V. it will feel 'splodgy', active or just particularly obvious. If the I.C.V. is operating normally it will feel firm, positive and responsive. In Gentle Touch™ Reflexology there are three key areas that can indicate levels of stress.

These are:

🦶 The Ileo-Caecal Valve (ICV)

🦶 The Solar Plexus

🦶 The Temporomandibular Joint (TMJ)

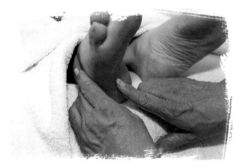

Colon (Large Intestine)

In a tiny baby it is very hard to specifically locate the individual sections of the colon. Working over and through the appropriate areas is acceptable, as all areas relating to the bowels and intestines will have been worked. In this way your thumbs will have covered all the necessary areas, as it is harder to know exactly where each area starts and stops on a small child's foot.

The following relates to the various sections that may be identified in a child of about six years upwards.

The reflex areas for the colon and small intestines are in a curve that starts on the right foot (on your left) and continues onto the left foot (on your right). This particular technique flows from one foot onto the other and it is important to work in the direction, as specified.

🖎 The bowel starts at the Ileo Caecal Valve (ICV) and moves up the arch of the foot / palm of the hand. It continues across the middle to the other foot / hand, where it goes across, down and around – see image.

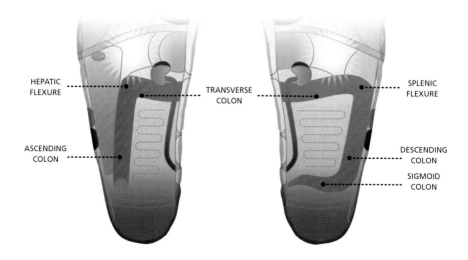

HEPATIC FLEXURE   TRANSVERSE COLON   SPLENIC FLEXURE

ASCENDING COLON   DESCENDING COLON   SIGMOID COLON

Ascending Colon to Hepatic Flexure

 Follow the ascending colon up from the I.C.V (on the right foot) towards the liver. Work around the edge of the liver to the hepatic flexure. Work up using one thumb following the other.

Transverse Colon

 Move from the hepatic flexure and work along (horizontally) across to the medial aspect (middle) of the right foot. Hold the point mid-way along the transverse colon on the medial aspect (inside edge) of the right foot and pick it up at the same level on the left foot. See image

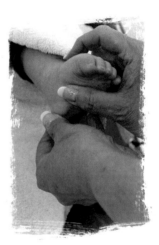

Work across the transverse colon, using the right thumb, until you reach the Splenic flexure (the 'corner' of the colon by the spleen in left foot).

Descending Colon / Sigmoid Colon

Always work in the direction described above, as the intention is to assist the child to be able to process everything in a healthy manner. This includes the correct passage and flow of faeces. Work the direction one way, without sweeping backwards and forwards.

 Work down (vertically) the descending colon from the Splenic flexure to the same level as the I.C.V.. Turn and loop across to the left, towards the rectum on the medial aspect. The descending colon becomes the sigmoid colon at the same level as the I.C.V. The sigmoid colon dips down from right to left (of the left foot) before slightly rising again towards the left side of the same foot (the rectum and the anus). See image

The bowels, in good condition, will feel uniform, responsive and smooth. Irregularity such as heat, lumps, bumps etc. can indicate an imbalance. Work and repeat as necessary. Follow with the bowel sweep if desired, (see Optional Extra on page 78)

Small Intestines

🦶 The small intestine is on the main area of the arch of the foot / palm area of the hand.

Using gentle thumb movement and pressure, work across the area under the arch of the foot / palm of the hand. Work horizontally; progressively moving downwards. Be careful not to go over the large bowel area again.

Bladder / Ureter / Kidneys (Right foot / hand)

The bladder, ureter and kidney reflex areas are as shown in the image on the next page.

The simplest way to encourage the function and flow from kidneys to bladder, and onto excretion, is to gently run your thumb down the arch of the foot, close to the inside edge (medial aspect). See image

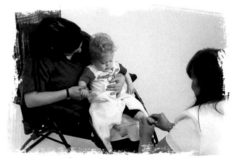

Children will often need to visit the toilet following a treatment of 'The Gentle Touch Reflexology™'. Babies may need an extra nappy / diaper change shortly after the treatment as it can increase the function and activity of the kidneys and increase production of urine.

 Place the flat of the thumb on the puffy area below the spine. This 'sack like' area is the reflex point for the bladder. Turn your thumb to point upwards on the underneath of the foot. Follow up just to the left of the side of the foot for the ureter, and hence to the kidney. The kidney floats around and is felt in many different locations. Generally, it can be found immediately below the transverse colon and directly above the ureter. Work extremely lightly up to the kidney and then smooth down towards the bladder. This is important to help 'flush' the baby / child's system and eliminate waste products.

Sciatic Line / Pelvis

🖐 The reflex point for the sciatic nerve is a line going across the heel of both feet

🖐 The reflex area for the pelvis is the heel area

🖐 On the hands the reflex point for the pelvis is a line worked across the heel of the hand. This is also the sciatic line.

Use your thumbs to apply a firm pressure and work across the sciatic line. This is immediately below the line separating the arch of the foot from the heel. The heel area of the foot / hand is generally slightly lighter or pinker in colour and much firmer to touch. In the foot this is the actual location of the sciatic nerve, as it runs down the legs and into the feet.

Continue working the rest of the heel area with a double thumb bounce, either vertically or horizontally. This completes the reflex points for the pelvic region on the underside of the foot / hand.

Repeat on the left foot / hand; intestines, bladder, kidney, sciatic and pelvis.

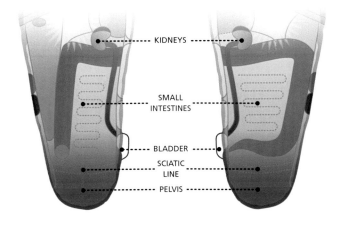

Ovaries / Testes (Right foot)

🖎 The reflex points for the ovaries / testes are on the outside (lateral aspect) of both feet / hands. It is only a very small area underneath the ankle / wrist bone and will probably only be felt if there is a problem.

Lymphatic Drainage (Groin)

🖎 The reflex areas for the lymphatic drainage points in the groin are situated around the ankle bone or wrist area on the hands.

Begin with a smooth, gentle 'finger ripple walk', starting at the outside of the ankle bone and moving up onto the top of the foot. From there sweep down to, and around the ankle bone. Repeat these moves working up the foot / hand, until the last sweep is under the toes / fingers.

This technique may assist the circulation and function of both the circulatory system and encourage general lymphatic drainage. This aids the elimination of waste products and supports the immune system.

Repeat on the left foot / hand - Lymphatic Drainage (Groin)

Complete the treatment at this stage by either:

🖎 Additional work on any vulnerable reflex points or areas

🖎 A further gentle rock into the Solar Plexus.

🖎 Optional Extra techniques. (see page 78)

Closing the Treatment

Smooth both of the feet / hands and close the treatment by holding your hands just slightly over the top of the foot / hands. This is called the Energy Cap. It can be done for a few seconds or longer, as desired. Make a conscious thought to disconnect from the treatment and the baby / child. Then wrap their feet / hands in a towel.

Acknowledge that during the time of the treatment you gave your best and aim to stay positive afterwards.

Do not worry about the baby / child after that. Remember that energy follows thought so if you worry it is not helpful to the baby / child.

Give of your best and be ready to treat again another time.

> **Important Reminder:** Get into the habit of thinking about a baby's / child's feet in terms of their organs, systems or body part locations.

 Reflexology Practitioners: Remember to write up your full treatment notes of everything that you found, key points of the treatment, responses and suggestions, and affected reflex areas that you may wish to assess at the next treatment.

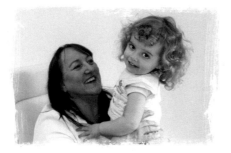

Optional Extra Techniques

The Cuddle

This is perhaps one of the most penetrating and exceptionally simple of all the techniques. The correct application of this technique can produce rewarding results. It is especially appropriate for anyone needing tender loving care, affection, support and contact. Everyone will benefit from the application of the cuddle. It is really the same as giving the child an all encompassing hug!

Place one hand under the foot; along the ball of the foot, (lung reflexes). Ensure that your fingers are along the line of the toes. Rest your other hand on top of the foot, (chest area) and slightly crossed with the other hand. Gently use a little pressure and rotate both hands. When treating an older child you may need to move your chair to the right of the child. You need to be almost at the side of them in order to be able to treat in an effective and relaxed manner. Allow yourself to join in with the soothing, almost rocking motion, and let the action flow!

Bowel Sweep

The bowel sweep is particularly useful for children who have bowel irregularities, including constipation.

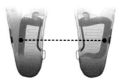

Start by placing your left hand on top of the right foot and oil the hand using the middle of your hands as an ink well. Oil your right thumb and smooth it along the line of the colon. Initially oil along ascending colon and transverse on right foot and when sufficiently oiled, smooth along the line of the colon with flat of right thumb. Finish with oiling along the transverse, descending and sigmoid colon on left foot. Sweep along the whole of the bowel line with your right thumb and then repeat this technique two or three times. It is a very soothing and effective for bowel conditions.

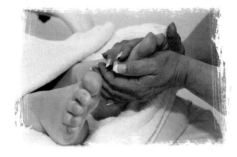

Making a Difference

"My Son has ADHD and I found that his Reflexology treatments have made a great difference. We have noticed that he is much calmer and more focused."

Mother L

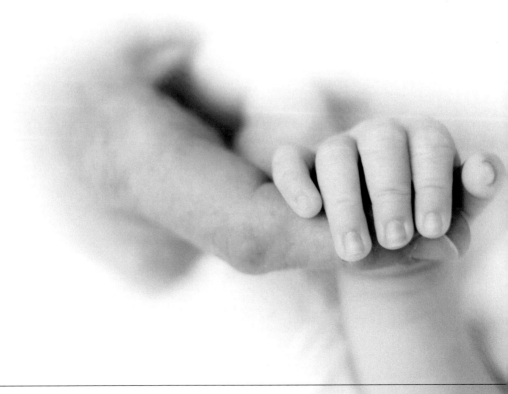

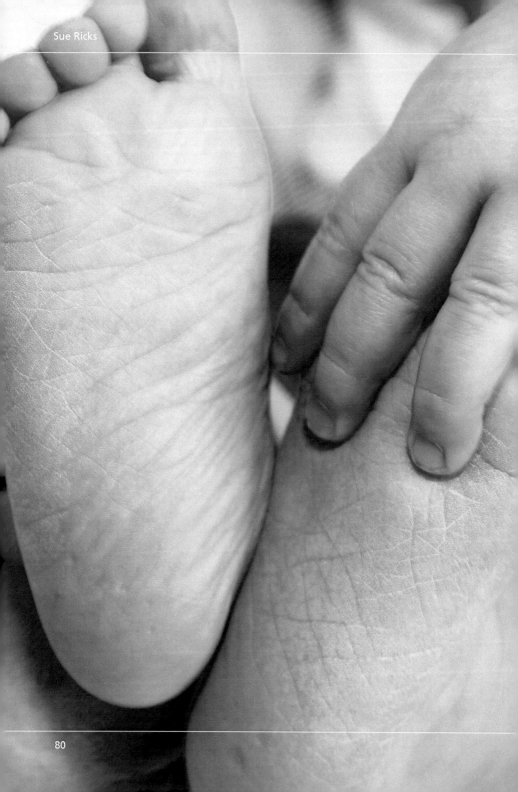

Conditions

Always remember to focus on the child e.g. "Sam is experiencing colic today" rather than "the baby always gets colic".

Twelve of the most commonly encountered conditions that a child may be experiencing.

1. Asthma

2. Colic (Wind)

3. Constipation

4. Crying

5. Diarrhoea

6. Earache

7. Eczema

8. Relaxation

9. Sinus congestion (Snuffles!)

10. Sleep

11. Teething

12. Vomiting / Reflux

1. Asthma

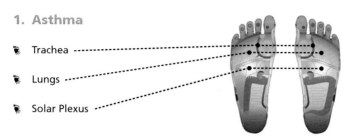

🦶 Trachea

🦶 Lungs

🦶 Solar Plexus

Mild cases only

Stimulating and relaxing the respiratory systems can alleviate the symptom of Asthma. Asthma can cause great levels of anxiety that can aggravate the condition. Reflexology will assist the relaxation of the whole person whilst assisting the whole bronchial area. Work down and around the big toe from the top to the bottom of the ball of the big toe. Gently work the area of the lungs (across the ball of the foot) and ease gently into the solar plexus. Also work slowly down the trachea reflex area to connect with the lungs. Gently and lightly, double thumb 'bounce' down the lung reflex areas and then smooth up again. Begin at lateral edge (outer / shoulder reflex) and work across the ball of the foot by working down and then smoothing up. Continue to work steadily towards the medial aspect. Stop at the natural line / crease around the ball of the big toe joint.

2. Colic (Wind)

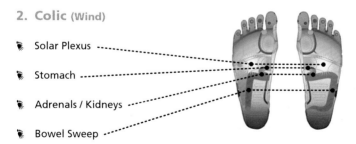

🦶 Solar Plexus

🦶 Stomach

🦶 Adrenals / Kidneys

🦶 Bowel Sweep

Working the reflexes for the pelvis and hips will encourage flow and slight movement of the hips. The gentle rotation of the hips can also provide an internal massage of the internal organs and digestive tract. Gentle easing into the solar plexus with soothing bowel sweeps.

3. Constipation

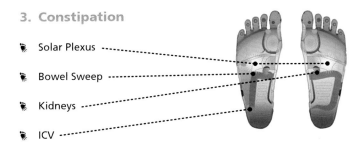

- Solar Plexus
- Bowel Sweep
- Kidneys
- ICV

Check for healthy hydration levels and encourage monitoring of water intake. Dehydration is one of the main reasons for constipation. Also check for sugar levels in formula milk, juices and medicines. Gentle easing into the solar plexus with soothing bowel sweeps and lightly smooth through the digestive system.

4. Crying

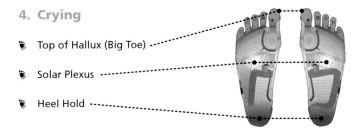

- Top of Hallux (Big Toe)
- Solar Plexus
- Heel Hold

Work sensitively by resting your thumbs on or over the solar plexus. Your thumbs may seem bigger than the baby's foot. However, if you work very lightly, you can get a soothing result. Keep repeating this gentle technique and stay calm. Speak reassuringly, calmly and quietly to the child. The child will pick up your energy and remain relaxed. Continue relaxing into the solar plexus and making gentle sweeping movements (as described earlier) for as long as is necessary.

5. Diarrhoea

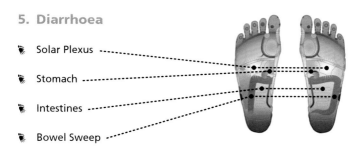

🐾 Solar Plexus

🐾 Stomach

🐾 Intestines

🐾 Bowel Sweep

Work sensitively by resting your thumbs gently on the solar plexus. Ensure quiet, slow and restful movements from the intestines through the colon. Dehydration can be a serious issue, so seek medical advice if necessary.

Diarrhoea may also be as a result of intolerance to dairy products.

A friend was concerned about her baby when he was little as he always had runny nappies. Luckily she found out that an intolerance to dairy products may be the cause. She changed her son's diet and he is fine now.

6. Earache

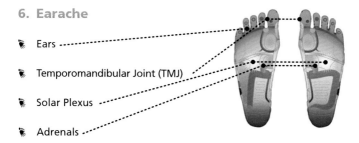

🐾 Ears

🐾 Temporomandibular Joint (TMJ)

🐾 Solar Plexus

🐾 Adrenals

One of the most common causes of earache and ear infections, including loss of hearing, is actually caused by an intolerance to dairy products. There is a great deal of information available on this subject including 'Are you a baby cow?' on www.suericks.com

Work the Temporomandibular Joint (TMJ) and ear reflexes, either side of the base of the fourth toes. Hold the side of the Big Toe (hallux) at the level of the joint and move in a rotational action when working the TMJ.

7. Eczema

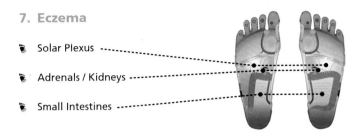

❧ Solar Plexus ----........

❧ Adrenals / Kidneys --------------

❧ Small Intestines ----------------

The skin represents the barrier between us and our surroundings. Eczema is another condition that can be exacerbated by dairy intolerance. (See personal Account on page 93)

Place your thumbs on the solar plexus to calm and relax the child. Eczema can also really flare up if the child gets agitated. Work through the bowel reflex points to assist the absorption of nutrients. Rest your thumbs over the kidney / adrenals to still any over-activity.

8. Relaxation

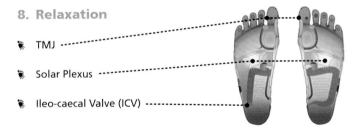

❧ TMJ ---------------

❧ Solar Plexus ------------------

❧ Ileo-caecal Valve (ICV) ----------------------

Very gentle easing into the solar plexus will aid relaxation. Use two fingers either side of the TMJ to relax this area. It also relates to skeletal and energetic balance. Work the ICV gently to support the function of this sensitive location. It is the physical location that prevents backflow of the digested material in the intestines / colon. The quality of the ICV represents the ability to cope with 'digesting' what is going on around oneself.

9. Sinus congestion (snuffles!)

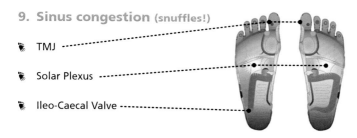

* TMJ

* Solar Plexus

* Ileo-Caecal Valve

Babies and children can frequently get discomfort resulting from sinus congestion and catarrh. They can be 'snuffly' and experience nasal discomfort when:

* Teething

* Have colds

* Have viruses

Work the top of the toes (pads) gently in a circular motion and then drain down the toes.

10.   Sleep

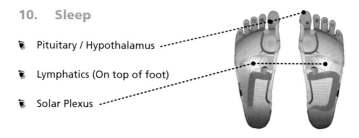

* Pituitary / Hypothalamus

* Lymphatics (On top of foot)

* Solar Plexus

Pay attention to both of the locations for the pituitary and hypothalamus. The pituitary area is at the centre of the swirls of the big toe and also at the top of the toe (Hallux).

The pituitary works intensively during growth and development. In babies / children the melatonin / serotonin cycles have not yet fully developed (sleep / wake cycles). Balancing the pituitary and hypothalamus can be relaxing.

11. Teething

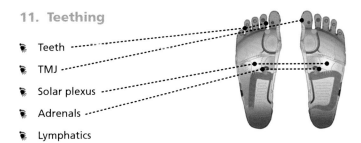

* Teeth
* TMJ
* Solar plexus
* Adrenals
* Lymphatics

Gently press the Solar Plexus, rotate the Temporomandibular Joint (TMJ) and then drain the lymphatics. Drain up the lymphatic channels (the gaps between the metatarsals), using right and / or left finger(s). Begin at the mid-line of the foot and work up to the toes. The reflex points for the teeth are mid-way down the sides of each toe.

There is also a reflex area that relates to the whole jaw and this can be found across the joint of the hallux (dorsal aspect - top of the toe). Working down the sides of the toes or as closely as possible (if there is room) can often bring relief. Sometimes with tiny babies it is sufficient to run your fingers over the tops of all the toes and also work round the side of the little toe.

12. Vomiting / Reflux

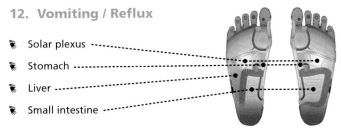

* Solar plexus
* Stomach
* Liver
* Small intestine

Check for common causes:-

* Feeding too fast
* Swallowing too much wind
* Ingesting while lying too flat (air gets trapped by diaphragm)
* Mother (if feeding) or child has eaten something indigestible or that they are intolerant to

Soothe the stomach reflex area by resting your thumbs on the stomach reflex points, this will reduce anxiety by gently working the solar plexus.

Children with Special Needs

Reflexology can be the best possible form of connection with a child with special needs. I have worked in many areas and found that children can really access some positive things with this form of therapy. The treatment allows for those caring for the child to use touch to access the spirit and essence of the child in a unique way. This may be one way that really allows for a special connection to take place and for a form of rapport to be built on to allow other forms of interaction to take place. Some children can be very private, in their own world. The application of this therapeutic touch can bring some great results. Always explain what the treatment will be like, what you will be doing and respect the child's connection to the treatment. They may take some time to be comfortable or to get used to it.

Some children find social interaction harder and may need familiar routines i.e. children diagnosed with Autism or Aspergers Syndrome. A very short treatment of the basic reflex areas is highly recommended for these cases. The treatment can be extended later if the child is happy to allow it to continue. They may become more generally settled and may show enjoyment, appreciation or acceptance of the treatments. This can bring joy to parents and carers who have a new way of connecting with the child in a shared realm of treatments.

Children who have sensory loss also greatly appreciate the sense of caring touch and so Gentle Touch™ Reflexology can help them connect with people in a new way. It can also help the child to release any pent up feeling or frustrations. Many parents report that their children are calmer, contented or seem happier. There are so many different ways in which a child may have special needs but the core abilities of reflexology is about accessing the inner person and supporting them through life's journey. This is the same for a child with learning or living challenges as it is for a fit and healthy child. Every person (young or old) deserves the same care, love, touch and kindness. The gentle touch of reflexology can be just that.

> The gentle and quiet touch of these treatments can bring joy and rewards to both the giver and receiver.

General Technique – Grounding Touch

Just cupping your hands around the child's feet is one of the most supportive and helpful techniques. Gently hold both of the heels of the child for as long as you feel is necessary. This can be a few seconds to perhaps a minute, whatever feels right. Trust your intuition.

The Role of a Reflexology Practitioner

Quite simply, I believe that this to act as a facilitator

It is the child themselves that does the healing. It is up to the practitioner to do the best job that they can but we really are facilitators for their own healing. The care that they receive through having their Reflexology treatment is part of what they are doing to take care of themselves, and also part of a care team's package of love and support. Offer the best treatment possible and that hopefully will assist the baby or child to be able to do their own individual healing. It is not possible to push anything into the body or 'make' anything happen. A Reflexologist facilitates the healing process by doing a treatment that can help him / her towards doing what their own body wishes to do. It maybe needs support or literally a helping hand along the way. Not everything is possible and however hard we try there are some things that are not meant to be. As long as everyone does their best, then offering Reflexology to a child will assist them as much as is practical or possible. We can never guarantee any outcomes.

Studies have shown that a loving touch can make a remarkable difference to people under stress and so when a Reflexologist works on the corresponding reflex points this helps to activate the innate healing responses in the body and also provides 'a helping hand'. This is one of the factors that assist the child with their own way of healing. This might be a much more authentic way to acknowledge the role of the Reflexologist as a facilitator. The alternative is to think that the only way someone can heal, is to continue to visit, or be visited by, a Reflexologist.

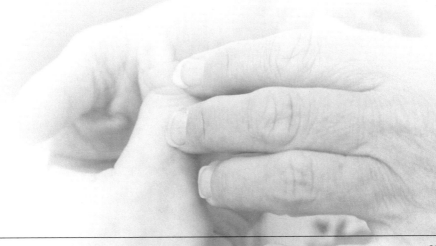

Deciding when to give advice and guidance (or not!)

You can decide for yourself if you will just perform a treatment or if you will offer additional advice and insights according to your observations. When providing additional information it may be useful to check if this supplementary support is requested, required or desired.

If they want to know about something then there is a better chance of them hearing the information and reacting to the suggestions made.

One way to check if they really want to know is to tell the person that there may be some additional information on this subject and ask "would you like to know?" Their response, and noticing how they react, will tell you whether they may really want to know.

They may be:

* Being polite when they say "yes"

* Do not want to know (at this time)

* Do not think it applies to them

* Think that they know it already, so do not need to hear it again

* It's not relevant to them

People generally do not receive unsolicited advice well!
Check to see if the information that you may wish to share is required.

Biggest Smile

"My baby was suffering from wind and pain in her tummy. Her responses during Sue's treatment were amazing and she smiled her biggest smile following the session! She has been more contented and smiley since, and I would definitely recommend Sue's treatment to any parents with babies suffering any discomfort."

Mother R

Dairy Intolerance

If a child is experiencing any prolonged or repeated symptoms of:

- Blocked sinuses
- Facial pressure around their sinuses
- Ear aches
- Hearing loss
- Repeated infections, including throat and ear

These could be a signal that a baby's / child's body is trying to tell them that it is not coping with the milk products in their food.

There are also other ways in which dairy intolerance can show up, these include:

- Headaches
- Nasal congestion
- Poor hearing
- Rogue "tummy" aches
- Repeated colds, throat infections, tonsillitis
- Snoring
- Aching
- Eczema
- Diarrhea

All of these are especially noticeable in children and yet also common in adults.

If a child is experiencing symptoms that are aggravated by dairy products then checking labels for the following can be helpful:

- Milk or milk derivatives
- Casein
- Lactose
- Whey

If you suspect that this could be an issue it is advisable to seek further professional advice and guidance, as well as checking out other available information i.e. the internet.

My Family Experience – Eczema / Dairy

I have personal experience of this as my own grandson was put onto steroids when he was diagnosed with Eczema at the age of 5 months. He was prescrlbed bathing products and steroid creams that were applied every day. Everything came to a head when his loving parents questioned why he screamed so much every time he was bathed and 'creamed'. My son had asked my opinion and I had shared my thoughts on a possible aggravation, but he was understandably following his doctors and consultant advice.

One night it was so bad they decided to put him onto another diary free formula and ask the health visitor for an appointment to discuss his inflamed skin condition. Three days later they saw the health visitor and explained what they had done, wanting to check her opinion. The evidence was clear to see as their son had totally clear skin!

The health visitor was amazed and said she had heard of this but thought it was impossible. She suggested putting their son back onto dairy products to see if he reacted as badly again. If so, that would be sufficient proof to get the formula required on prescription (free in the UK). They did not want to put their son through that misery again, so they have decided to pay for the formula themselves.

They have been surprised at the variety of responses from professionals, friends and family to the changes in his skin condition. Luckily they had access to information that enabled them to make their own informed decision and are convinced that they have done the right thing for their son. They have now found a very knowledgeable, aware and supportive health visitor.

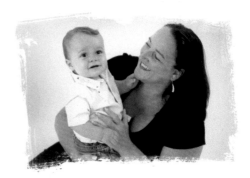

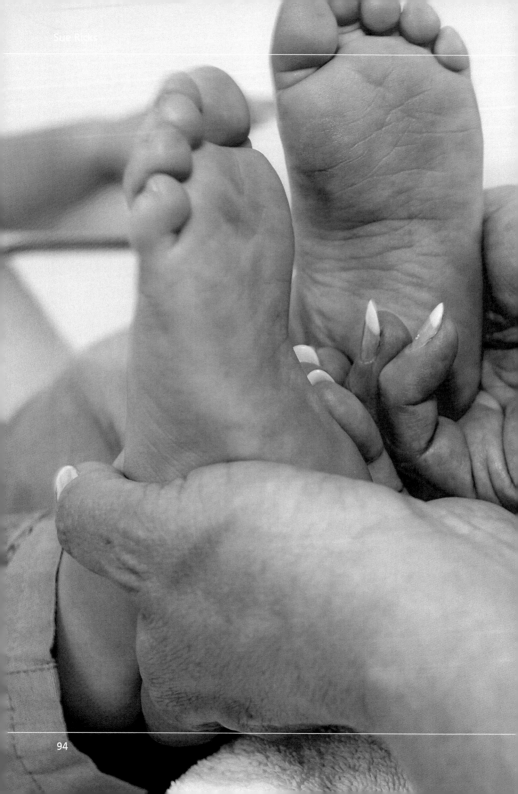

Children's Feet

It is essential that everyone takes care of children's feet and the action of taking a child for Reflexology is one way of paying healthy attention to the child's feet. Being aware of your child's feet is as important as being aware of their medical health, or taking them to the dentist for regular check-ups.

Reflexologists can be the first line in noticing that something may need extra attention. Children with any abnormalities should be referred to a medical practitioner or a podiatrist, who will be able to assess the degree of severity and advise on possible exercises or braces required, to correct issues in the early stages.

The human foot is a very complicated part of the body and the feet of young children are soft and pliable. Any abnormal pressures can easily cause the foot to deform. The foot of a child grows rapidly during the first year, reaching almost half their adult foot size. That first year can be very important in the development of the feet.

A Calming Touch

"My baby cried from the moment that he emerged. He seemed angry and upset from the word go. My friend is a reflexologist and she seemed to be able to calm him just by touching his feet. I have no idea how it works but work it does!"

Mother K

What is normal and what is abnormal?

Luckily it is not as normal for children to experience foot pain or deformities due to the flexibility and resilience of a child's foot. Assessing is the role of the medically trained professionals.

Common issues

Athlete's Foot - Tinea pedis

Athlete's foot is caused by a parasitic fungus and is a communicable disease (transmittable to others). It can be transmitted by sharing footwear, sharing towels with someone who has Athlete's foot, and in moist environments where people walk barefoot.

These include;

- Showers
- Sports centre
- Changing rooms
- Swimming baths

The same fungus that causes Athlete's foot can also cause skin conditions elsewhere:

- Toenails - (Onychomycosis)
- Groin - (tinea curries)

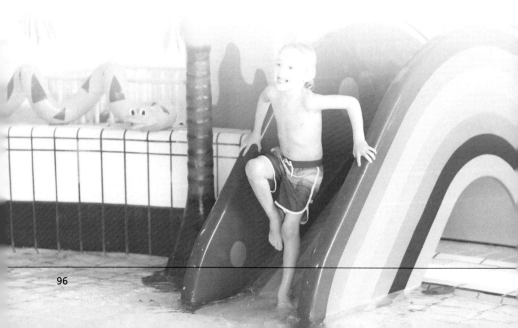

Smelly Feet - Bromodis

The feet have more sweat glands than any other part of the body.

Advice is to:

- Wash the feet thoroughly twice daily

- Dry the feet carefully, especially between the toes

- Apply foot (not body) lotion

- Make sure that shoes have dried out between uses

- Change socks regularly

Also drink more water to hydrate the body and assist healthy sweat production as dehydration, hormonal changes, anxiety and certain medications can affect the quantity and quality of the sweat released by the feet.

Warts and Verrucas

Warts are generally found on the hands or other areas of the body. Verrucas are found on feet and are otherwise called 'plantar warts'. They are caused by the HPV (human papilloma virus). These can be spread from one person to another via contact with a contaminated surface or through close skin contact. Verrucas and warts are more likely to be spread if the skin is damp, wet or damaged.

Ideally the immune system will reject and overcome the virus and the warts and verrucas drop off. They can last for a short or long while (from weeks to months or even years). They can also drop off literally overnight.

Warts don't cause any harm however some children find them itchy, painful or simply embarrassing. Verrucas however are more likely to be painful. This can feel uncomfortable or tender, like standing on a needle.

The reason they are painful is because HPV causes a hard protein called keratin that is in the top layer of the skin (the epidermis) to grow too much. This produces the rough or hard texture of a wart or verruca.

If a child has a verruca it is recommended to cover it with a plaster before doing any reflexology to avoid any cross contamination. Gloves are an alternative option for these cases or those of athletes foot.

Toe Nails

Damaged nails

The most common injury to a toe nail is from bruising after stubbing the toe, or dropping something on it. It can take a month for a toe nail to come off, and another year for it to grow back again. It can also be caused by wearing inappropriate foot wear or extensive exercise. This is often found in long distance runners.

Infected nails

These will start to crumble around the edges and may be yellow in colour.
The surrounding area may also be inflamed. The commonest cause is T. rubrum which also causes Athlete's foot.

Some of the natural remedies for toenail fungus include:

- Using Tea Tree Oil on and around the toenail

- Grapefruit Seed Extract is also known to have antimicrobial activity

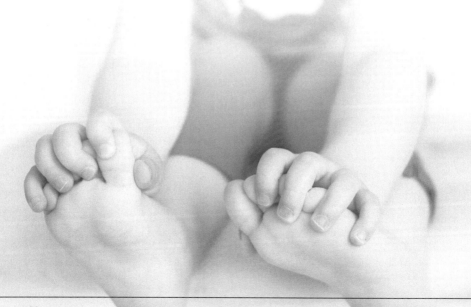

Psoriatic nails

Reddening around the edges of the nails or yellowing can be as a result of psoriasis, but is much less likely in children.

Ingrowing toe nails

An ingrown toenail (onychocryptosis) occurs when part of the nail penetrates the skin, which can often result in an infection. The ingrown nail can also apply pressure in the nail fold area without penetrating the skin - this is not technically an ingrown toe nail, but can also be painful. A corn / callus is also common down the side of the nail and is a reaction to this pressure, rather than the nail actually penetrating the skin.

Ingrowing toe nails may represent 'ingrowing' or 'painful' thoughts. Ingrowing toe nails can coincide with times of deep thoughts that are painful. The deeper the toe nail is pressing (or infected), the deeper the thoughts.

Some Nail Facts

- Toe nails grow faster in the summer than they do in the winter

- Toe nails grow at the same speed on both feet (however if you are right handed then the nails on your right hand will grow quicker than your left!)

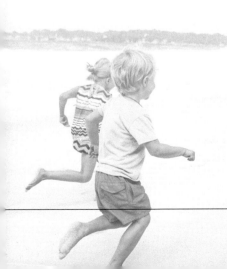

Prevention

Keeping Healthy Feet and Toe Nails

- Keep feet clean and dry

- Have feet measured professionally

- Wear shoes that are suitable for the job and are well fitting

- Only wear own shoes (do not share)

- Wear waterproof sandals in shower rooms or locker rooms

- Wear socks inside shoes and only wear once before washing

- Never wear tight shoes

- Inspect toe nails for damage or sensitivity

- Keep nails trimmed

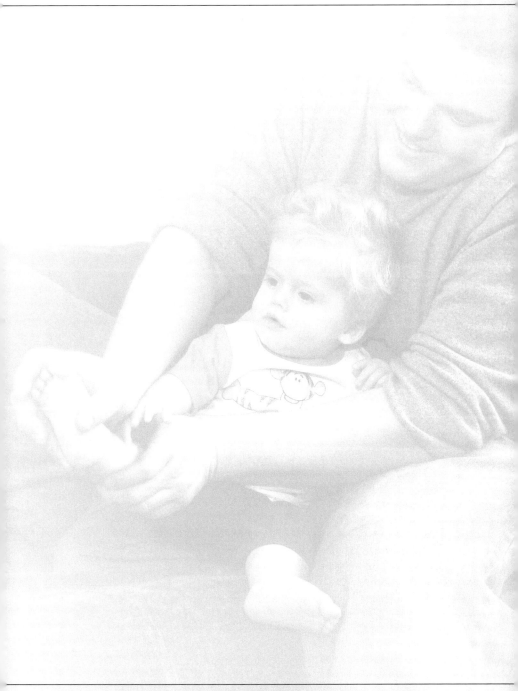

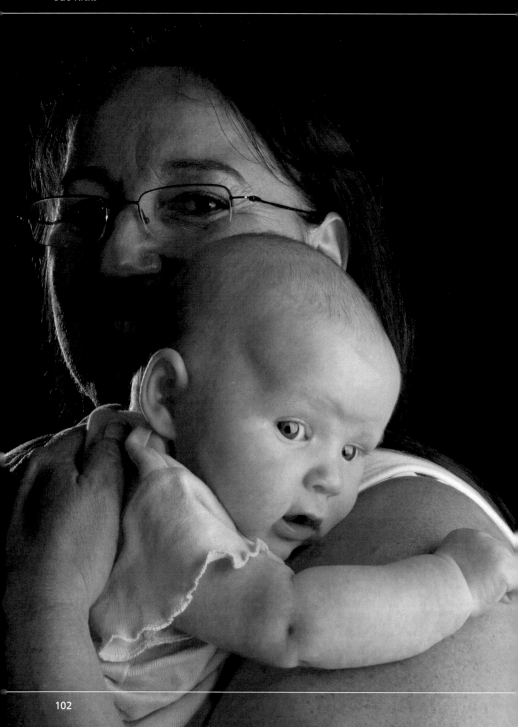

Useful Information

There are numerous factors that can make a difference when working with babies and children. It is useful to know about, or be aware of, a range of issues. I have found that frequently the simplest and smallest shifts can make the biggest difference to a child's health and happiness.

Nutrition and Food Awareness

Nutritional Bonus

Avoiding Toxins and Protecting Tender Young Skin

Avoiding Geopathic Stress (harmful earth rays)

Bed Wetting

Care Over Sleeping Areas and Desk Placement

Rest and Relaxation

Talking with Children

Chakra Information

Alternative Meanings

Professional Considerations

Nutrition and Food Awareness

It is now common knowledge that it is important to feed a child quality and nourishing food. What may not be discussed is **how** that food is cooked!

Microwaves

Methods of cooking also impact on the value of the food content. Avoid microwave cooking as this depletes the energetic value of the food. Additionally, the effect of the microwaving action does not stop once the food is inside the child's body. The agitation (friction) of molecules that causes the heat continues. The soft internal tissue can also be affected.

Many mothers may express their breast milk and then freeze it for their babies' future use. This breast milk is then either thawed, or warmed in the microwave. This destroys any of the essential energy remaining. This is such a great shame when the mother has gone to so much effort to provide what she believes to be the very best for her child. Heating or thawing human milk destroys it's protective antibodies, even at low temperatures. Warming breast milk in a microwave destroys 98% of its immunoglobulin-A antibodies and 96% of it's liposome activity. It also reduces the milk's resistance to the highly infectious E Coli bacteria.

Dr Lita Lee stated in the Lancet 9th Dec 1989.
"Microwaving Baby formulas converted certain trans-amino acids into their synthetic cis-isomers. Synthetic isomers, whether cis-amino acids or trans-fatty acides, are not biologically active. Further, one of the amino acids, L-proline, was converted to its d-isomer which is known to be neurotoxic (poisonous to the nervous system) and nephrotoxic (poisonous to the kidneys.) It's bad enough that many babies are not nursed, but now they are given fake milk (baby formula) made even more toxic via microwaving."

So, warmed baby formula produces an entirely new amino acid that is toxic to the baby. There is also a significant risk of scalding after the use of microwaves. It is far safer to warm frozen or chilled milk in a bowl of warm / hot water.

Nutritional Bonus

Many children are quite picky about what they eat. Some children may get all the nutrition they need, and yet, for others, they choose or are provided with nutritionally inadequate food. Sadly many responsible parents and carers are unaware that the efforts they go to, in order to provide good food, may be hampered at source. It is a sad fact that some foods are produced in such a way that the essential mineral and vitamin content may be seriously depleted. The food looks good but is 'empty' of quality. This nutritional depletion can lead to signs, symptoms and behaviours that indicate a wide range of problems including Attention Deficit Disorder (ADD) or Attention Deficit Hyperactivity Disorder (ADHD).

I have worked closely with a specialist tutor at the Learn Write Centre, Long Eaton, Nottingham UK. We have found that numerous children benefit from the correct mineral and vitamin supplementation plus appropriate anti-oxidants and Omega 3's. (for more information contact suericks@suericks.com)

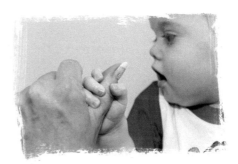

It is not possible to get the nutrients out of the ground if they are not in the ground in the first place! Modern intensive farming methods, cultivation, storage and sales demanded by so many supermarkets have had a direct effect on the depletion of the nutritional content of food. Locally grown, organic produce is the best option, if available. There are now many companies that deliver organic produce to your door.

Finding good quality food is not a new problem! As far back as 1936 the Senate Document number 264, stated that "sick soil means sick animals and sick people". In Victorian times the milk deliveries to cities were a two way process. The milk was transported into the cities and the clinker (soot from the chimneys) was carried back out on the empty carts and put back onto the fields; therefore enriching the soil and replacing lost minerals. Through an advancement of technology and modern times we have lost this essential cycle of replacing the minerals taken from the soil.

Avoiding Toxins and Protecting Tender Young Skin

An increasing number of parents, carers and grandparents, are becoming aware of the hidden dangers of normal everyday toiletries. I had assumed that if any ingredients were toxic or harmful in products, then companies would be stopped from using them. However I realise there was a great deal I did not know! Fortunately I have now had time to research the facts. Once we know the facts we can then decide on alternative action.

Medical researchers in the United States, Japan, Switzerland and Germany have produced evidence of how many toxic ingredients are in commonly used products, such as:

- Shampoos and 'baby' shampoos

- Shower gel and 'baby wash'

- Skin lotions and 'baby skin moisturisers'

- Baby and hygiene wipes

- Toothpaste, including junior or child toothpaste

Some of the constituents to be alert for include:

- Sodium Lauryl Sulphate (SLS)

- Sodium Laureth Sulphate (SLES)

- Propylene Glycol

- Talcum Power

Natural does not necessarily mean 'safe'. See information sheets at the end of this book for more information.

Searching out healthy alternatives can be essential for the benefit for children, for life.

Avoiding Geopathic Stress (harmful earth rays)

Babies and children are very sensitive to environmental and other energies. Many children are placed in their cot or bed and within a few hours are found to be either awake or have moved their position.

If a child is restless, unable to sleep, unwell or constantly moving position in bed / cot it is advisable to change the location of where they sleep. This can often alleviate the most traumatic of nights!

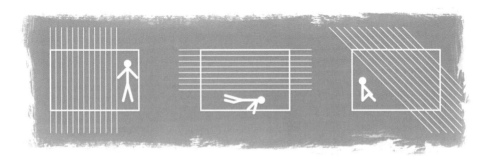

Bed Wetting

If a child is suffering due to bed-wetting it can sometimes be helpful to relocate the child's bed (see bed placement advice). Also do anything that you can to raise the child's esteem as it is such a common problem and can destroy their confidence. Generally children grow out of this, but there is a hidden stigma about it and it can be soul destroying for children coping with it. If a child is suffering, be practical and check any food sensitivities, including wheat and dairy products.

It is also recognised that there can be a hidden emotional content behind the bed wetting. A calming treatment before going to sleep can help a child settle into a comfortable sleep. There is also a suggestion that having treatments helps a child to become more bodily aware, as the treatments can trigger deep sensations in an individual. Some highly evolved children with deep sensitivities, also described by some as those "who have been here before", find that life is harsh and frightening and can be prone to bed wetting.

Care Over Sleeping Areas and Desk Placement

A few tips about where to place the essential furniture in a baby or child's bedroom or study area.

Avoid being in front of any corner (created by the corner of room or furniture).

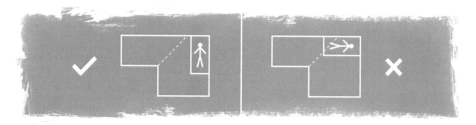

Avoid having the bed / cot directly in front of the door (sideways or angled is fine)

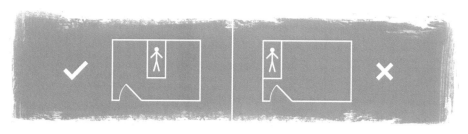

Avoid having a desk with the child's back to the window or door.
Keep mirrors or shiny reflective surfaces angled away from the sleeping area
(or cover mirrors / TV's etc at night). This can help to increase deeper sleep.

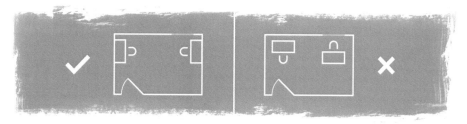

The energy flow that is unhelpful (inauspicious) is called a 'Sha Line' in Feng Shui. Sha lines are found at an angle of 45 degrees.

Baby with Neck Tension

"When I met Henry he could not move his neck to the left. He had been diagnosed with torticollis (neck tightness) by his pediatrician. I undertook the class in Gentle Touch ™ Reflexology two days before I treated him. I used the new way that I had learned to do the solar plexus connection and he was very sensitive to the touch. Initially he pulled away and yet as I continued to use the new approach and connect with him via his solar plexus, the tissue began to soften and ease. Very soon he turned his head to the left and looked at me. It was amazing. the mom said it was the first time she had seen him do that."

Michelle Emanuel
Occupational Therapist, CranioSacral Therapist,
Certified Infant Massage Instructor,
Cincinnati, OH, USA

Rest and Relaxation

Children, like adults, need time when they can switch off, and sometimes, they find it hard to do. Many may turn to the 'hypnotic attention seeker' – the TV, computer or games. This may be their way of being able to deal with their busy internal thoughts. A Reflexology session is a perfect way to calm a child, help them to relax and rebalance, without having to disappear into a game, television or computer. Children who have regular treatments find that they generally recover quicker from some of the most common ailments and illnesses. Not only does it help the child to recover from the illness but it also does not require any additional remedies – just hands or feet, or both!

Caring for a disabled child can be exhausting and yet often a very rewarding experience. The disruption to daily lives can be stressful. There can be an extensive workload to cope with. Reflexology can bring a breath of fresh air, time to relax, is easy to provide and can improve connection and 'bonding'! Many people talk about a shared time together during the treatment. One to one time can be invaluable. My experiences of working with disabled children have been that they generally view it very favourably, especially when it is fully explained and they understand what the potential benefits to themselves are. It is essential to give the child the rights over the treatment decisions, i.e. whether they want the treatment or not! I have found it to be incredibly helpful for children with both acute and chronic illnesses and challenges.

Talking with Children

It is essential that we say what we mean!

How often have you heard someone say "don't touch" or "don't shout!"
What is usually meant is – "keep your hands still" or "please be quiet".

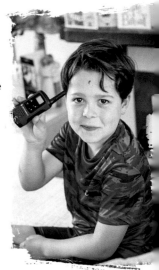

Children are very literal. When we say something, our brains follow the instruction quite literally.

For example – this simple instruction will illustrate the point. Instruction – Do NOT think about a purple and pink striped Zebra.

Did you think about it? – You probably did, even though you have been told not to. What about "Do NOT think about a rabbit on a trampoline" – did you think about it? - You probably did! Our brains delete the "do not" in the statement.

It is the same if we say "do not drop the cup" – the brain has to work out what that means i.e. how would we actually drop the cup. It means that our brains actually "pre-plan" how to drop the cup and therefore it becomes more likely that the person who heard that will probably drop the cup.

Be careful to only say what you actually mean and also help others to do the same. This important learning exercise opens far more effective styles of communication.

This applies to:

* Practitioners who are able to make themselves more clearly understood

* Parents as they connect with their children develop a better rapport through being able to communicate more effectively. This can greatly benefit their children too.

Examples:

Not Effective	Effective
Do not shout	Please be quiet
Don't forget your homework	Remember your homework
Don't leave your jacket on the floor	Please put your jacket away
Don't eat that with your fingers	Please use your knife and fork
That's not yours - give it back now	Please give that back to Kelly
You are not listening	Please listen to me

Motto – Say what you mean and what you want – not what you **DO NOT** want

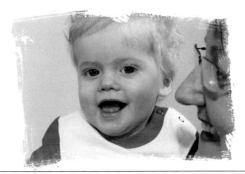

Chakra Information

There are increasing numbers of people who are interested in knowing more about human energy systems including Chakras. Understanding about chakras can help bring a new dimension to healing.

It can aid appreciation, understanding and knowledge of the whole person. It can help to understand their illnesses / conditions and reasons that may be behind their challenges.

The word 'Chakra' is a Sanskrit meaning 'wheel'. All of us have chakras. They are vortices within our energy system that help energies to flow in and around our bodies. When our chakras are in a healthy balance and alignment, then we feel happier, are healthier and have more vibrancy to enjoy life.

There are seven chakras (see chart)

All of the chakras rotate and can be thought of as energy pumping stations, as they move energy around our systems. Each chakra is like a wheel – a spinning vortex that acts like a funnel. It is the connection to the other dimensions of ourselves and our auras.

Front View   Side View

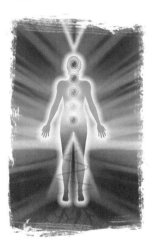
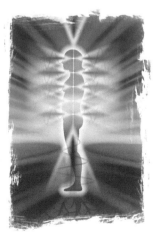

The seven main chakras:

Crown	Spiritual centre	Pineal	Purple
Brow	Intuition / Inner vision	Pituitary	Indigo, Blue (dark)
Throat	Communication / Self expression	Thyroid	Blue (light)
Heart	Love / Passion	Thymus	Green / Pink
Solar Plexus	Intellect / Logic	Pancreas	Yellow
Sacral / Splenic	Creativity / Processing	Adrenals	Orange
Base / Root	Grounding / Self preservation	Reproductive organs	Red

Four Key Points about each Chakra

(see chart on left page)

- A location, i.e. the Crown Chakra is a vortex found above the top of the head

- A related 'theme', i.e. the theme of the Brow Chakra is 'intuition'

- An Endocrine (hormonal) link, i.e. the Endocrine link for the Solar Plexus Chakra is the Pancreas

- An associated colour, i.e. the colour for the Base / Root Chakra is Red

Chakra Links to Body

The areas that the chakras 'govern', effect or link into are as follows:

Crown Chakra	Top of the head, upper scalp and head areas, pineal
Brow Chakra	Brow down to (and including), the maxilla (top of the mouth / jaw), pituitary, nose, eyes (perception), senses, upper teeth, nervous system (with solar plexus), ears, creative mind
Throat Chakra	Mandible (lower half of the mouth and jaw) and down to the area at the top of the sternum (breastbone), including the arms / hands, neck / shoulder and the top of the spine / lungs, throat, tonsils and tongue. Also the vocal cords, thyroid, parathyroid (bone density), bottom row of teeth, upper bronchii, upper areas of lungs, clavical, lower part of scapula
Heart Chakra	Heart, circulatory system, thymus gland (immune system) upper part of the sternum, lungs, heart, upper part of chest, rib cage, aorta and major arteries, thoracic spine. lower part of scapula
Solar Plexus Chakra	Lower part of chest, part of thoracic spine, stomach, pancreas, upper areas of intestines and colon (transverse), central nervous system, lower thoracic spine
Sacral Chakra	Kidneys, bladder (elimination), upper area of colon & intestines, upper lumbar spine, mid region of intestines and part of ascending and descending colon, reproductive organs
Root / Base Chakra	Legs, hips, feet, lower lumbar spine, bones in general, lower reproductive organs, lower areas of colon including sigmoid and rectum

The root / base, sacral and solar plexus are said to be the physical chakras whilst the heart, throat, brow and crown are the soul chakras.

The integration happens between the heart (soul) and the solar plexus (physical) and this why the area called the Solar Plexus is so important. It is where our body and soul connect.

The Aura and Chakras

The aura and chakras may sometimes be thought of as two separate things and yet they are actually part of each other. The aura is the energy field that emanates from in and around us. The chakras are part of the aura and are the means by which the physical body connects with the aura and vice versa. The vortex of the chakras connects with, and forms, part of the layers of the aura. The outer areas of the chakra vortices forms part of the aura and both interconnect with the other.

There are seven major chakras and many secondary ones in the palms of the hand, soles of the feet and also at major joints.

Physical problems may stem from emotional issues that are current or from the past. Knowledge of the chakras and what they relate to, can help when paying attention to what may be going on 'behind the scenes'. Sometimes the person is aware of the issue and sometimes they are unaware of it. In my work with both Reflexology and NLP (Neuro Linguistic Programming) I have become fascinated at how deep the links can go.

The connection between the physical body and chakra / auras is why it is helpful to work increasingly lightly over some reflex points.

Knowledge of the chakras can play an important part in the awareness of what a child may be experiencing and what potential contributing factors may be. The base and sacral chakras have a 'settling in' period when a child is born. When a baby is born 'naturally' it eases its way into the world via the Mother's base chakra, however when the baby is born via an assisted delivery (caesarean or forceps) the 'grounding' process can be hampered or interrupted. Ideally a baby's crown chakra enters their new physical world via the Mother's base chakra and a natural balancing occurs.

Balancing the Chakras

The seven energy centres can be brought into further balance by holding your thumb lightly over the top of the big toe (hallux) and rest a middle finger on the heal.

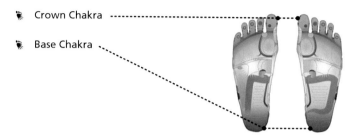

❧ Crown Chakra

❧ Base Chakra

Rest just a finger on each of these two points and 'wait' for the rebalancing to take place. Some practitioners may feel this balancing take place, whilst others may have to trust the process. A light and sensitive touch for 30 – 90 seconds can assist the balancing process. Anything done with the intention of balancing can be helpful.

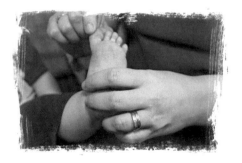

Alternative Meanings

| BLADDER | Ability to have control over body and functions
Holding on to / letting go
'Pissed' off? |

BOWELS / INTESTINES
Processing of nourishment.
Unsure what is good for them
Ability to absorb good things in life
Reflects relaxation vs stress
Diarrhoea – getting rid of quickly
Constipation – cannot let go (always remembers)
Trouble digesting life

BROKEN BONES
Time to 'break' with the old, and gain a "break-through"
Something had to "give"

CIRCULATION
Flow of blood / love around body

EAR PROBLEMS
Is there something that they don't want to hear / can't hear?
Difficulty in communication

EYE SIGHT PROBLEMS
What does the child find difficult to 'see'?
How do they feel about what they 'see'?
Chinese link to kidneys

GALL BLADDER
Decision making ability
Gall stones – fossilised ideas / energy / feelings

HAND / WRIST
Ability to 'handle' life / issues
Link to foot / ankle

HEAD
Thoughts / mind
Congestion = head full of thoughts
Emptiness = loss of energy exhausted
Possibly a Crown / Base chakra imbalance

HEADACHES
Needs love and attention – often giving
Leaves own thoughts / head depleted
Headaches – thoughts painful

HEART	Pumps love / blood around body and person
	Reflects heartfelt issues
HIPS	Pivot point
	Body connection to moving forward (also with knee)
	Fluidity / mobility
	Base / grounding
	Link to shoulder
KIDNEYS	House of fear
	Cleansing of body – Removes 'fear'
	Interlinked with adrenals and 'fright and flight'
	Chinese link to eyes
	Partnership issues – 2 kidneys in partnership
	Processing emotion
	(fluid = emotion. Kidneys keep fluid balance)
KNEES	Ability to move forward
	Link to elbow – ability to bend
LARGE INTESTINE	Unconscious thinking
	Chinese link to lungs
LIVER	Confidence
	Where have they been taking things to excess
	Ability to distinguish between good and bad / poisonous
LUNGS	Expression and inspiration
	It may be difficult to express feelings or take in
	Giving (out) and receiving (in) imbalance
	Chinese link to bowels
NAUSEA	What are you sick of?
	Refusal to accept
NECK	Connects head to body
	Allows us ability to look all around
	Allows variety of 'view points'
	May reflect ability / inability to cope with 'side' issues

PANCREAS	Balance of sugar / sweetness in life Unsatisfied desire for love / sweetness
PELVIS	Grounding 'Base' issues Crown / Base imbalance
SHOULDER	Shouldering all responsibilities and burdens Overburdened
SINUS CONGESTION	Withheld emotion Lots of thoughts that go round and round and are held onto Digestive imbalances – possible food intolerances Possible dairy produce sensitivity Mucal protection
SKIN	Barrier – Symbolizes line between self and exterior Rashes = irritation Boils = boiling over Related to touch and contact
SMALL INTESTINE	Links to brain – both absorb ideas / food Disorders = too analytical to absorb? Nothing 'hangs around' now = diarrhoea Conscious thinking
SPINE	Core of life What allows us to 'stand up to life' Are they getting the 'backing' they need?
SPLEEN	Energetic link to immune system Cleanser of blood / love
STOMACH	What can't they stomach? Is something eating them up?
TEMPOROMANDIBULAR JOINT = TMJ	One of three stress indicators (1 TMJ, 2 solar plexus, 3 ICV) Needed to masticate food & ingest food (take in goodness of life). Represents skeletal and energetic balance Tension – grinding teeth / grit your teeth and get on with it

Professional Considerations

If you are a practitioner working with babies and children you need to consider
the following:

1. Initial Consultation Notes / Case History Cards and Treatment Notes

* These must be written whilst being mindful that your client can ask to see anything that you have written

* All notes and client personal details must be protected by ensuring that you adhere to any Data Protection legislation that affects you

* All notes and client information must be stored in a safe manner so as to protect the information supplied to you by your clients and their children

* All dealings with your clients must be handled in a confidential manner (for more information on Confidentiality see 'Ten Things that you may not know about Confidentiality' – e-book available at www.suericks.com)

* Update client records for each visit

2. Regulations

Always check with your Local Council or Local Authorities for any regulations which may affect your Practice. Every area or region has its own laws, bye-laws and regulations so make sure that you find out what they are in your area, in case they affect your ability or permission to practice.

Be aware that different states / counties / countries allow or prohibit different things, so work with your professional bodies and find out if there are any specific laws etc. that affect what you do. In the UK there are a few curious ones like ensuring that anyone presenting with dental problems has to be referred to a dentist. This is probably a throwback to when anyone could whip teeth out for you! Regulations were created to protect us!

3. Medical Aid For Children Under 16

In the UK it is an offence for a parent or guardian to fail to provide medical aid for children under 16.

Treatments can be given, but only after medical care has been provided.

4. Conduct and Ethics

In the UK, the Association of Reflexologists (AoR) and the British Register of Complementary Practitioner (BRCP) require practitioners to follow Code of Conduct and Ethics. Check with your professional Associations for their regulations and codes of practice.

5. Insurance

Insurance is Vital – It is your duty to have appropriate insurance.

Note: If you switch insurers or cease trading you will need to check your policy regarding claims relating to the period of previous insurance i.e. run-off cover.

6. Trade Descriptions Act (UK) 1972

It is a criminal offence to falsely describe goods or services (either written or spoken), therefore be sensible and careful about how you describe what you do if you are treating children. Be careful to avoid words like cure, guarantee, promise etc.

7. Criminal Records Bureau (CRB Checks) - UK

Many sectors where you may be employed to work with children require a CRB check to be cleared before you can begin work. See their website for current legislation in UK.
www.crb.gov.uk

It is the responsibility of each person to check for legislation that may affect / impede their work.

Five Key Areas

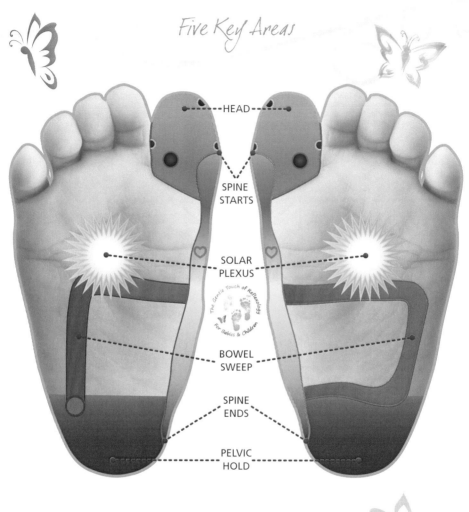

HEAD

SPINE
STARTS

SOLAR
PLEXUS

BOWEL
SWEEP

SPINE
ENDS

PELVIC
HOLD

BCRIA
The Babies & Children Reflexology
International Association
Approved Chart

Areas of the Spine

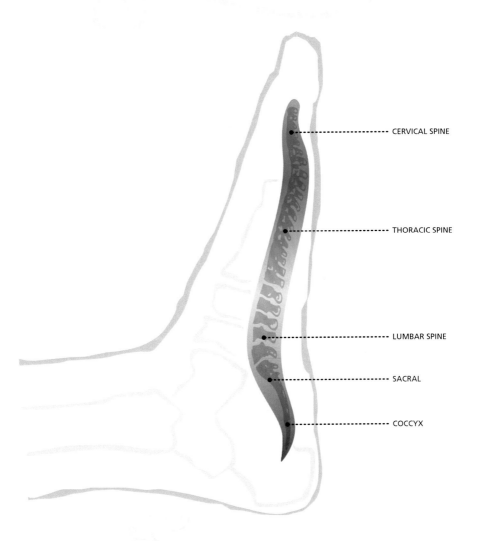

- - - - - - - - CERVICAL SPINE

- - - - - - - - THORACIC SPINE

- - - - - - - - LUMBAR SPINE

- - - - - - - - SACRAL

- - - - - - - - COCCYX

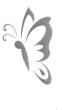

The Gentle Touch of Reflexology Foot Reflex Chart

GENTLE TOUCH ™ REFLEXOLOGY

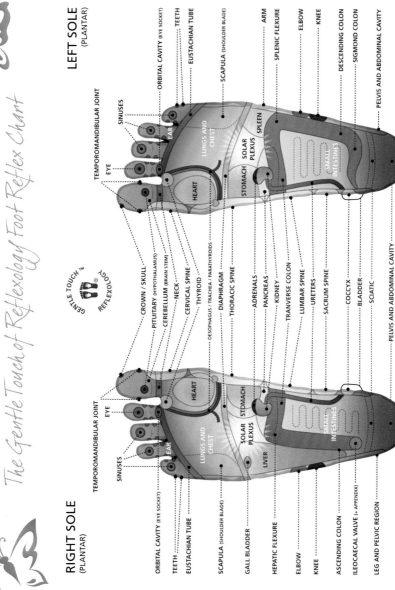

RIGHT SOLE
(PLANTAR)

LEFT SOLE
(PLANTAR)

RIGHT SOLE labels:
ORBITAL CAVITY (EYE SOCKET)
TEETH
EUSTACHIAN TUBE
SCAPULA (SHOULDER BLADE)
GALL BLADDER
HEPATIC FLEXURE
ELBOW
KNEE
ASCENDING COLON
ILEOCAECAL VALVE (+ APPENDIX)
LEG AND PELVIC REGION

TEMPOROMANDIBULAR JOINT
EYE
EAR
SINUSES

HEART
LUNGS AND CHEST
SOLAR PLEXUS
STOMACH
LIVER
SMALL INTESTINES

Centre column labels:
CROWN / SKULL
PITUITARY (HYPOTHALAMUS)
CEREBELLUM (BRAIN STEM)
NECK
CERVICAL SPINE
THYROID
OESOPHAGUS / TRACHEA / PARATHYROIDS
DIAPHRAGM
THORACIC SPINE
ADRENALS
PANCREAS
KIDNEY
TRANVERSE COLON
LUMBAR SPINE
URETERS
SACRUM SPINE
COCCYX
BLADDER
SCIATIC
PELVIS AND ABDOMINAL CAVITY

LEFT SOLE labels:
ORBITAL CAVITY (EYE SOCKET)
TEETH
EUSTACHIAN TUBE
SCAPULA (SHOULDER BLADE)
ARM
SPLENIC FLEXURE
ELBOW
KNEE
DESCENDING COLON
SIGMOND COLON
PELVIS AND ABDOMINAL CAVITY

TEMPOROMANDIBULAR JOINT
SINUSES
EYE
EAR

LUNGS AND CHEST
SPLEEN
SOLAR PLEXUS
STOMACH
HEART
SMALL INTESTINES

Gentle Touch™ Reflexology

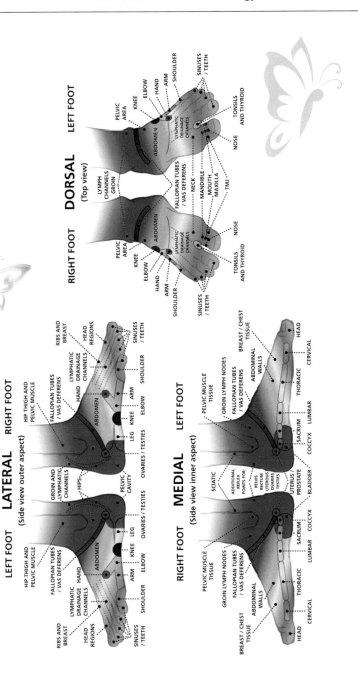

Gentle Touch™ Reflexology

The Gentle Touch of Reflexology Hand Reflex Chart

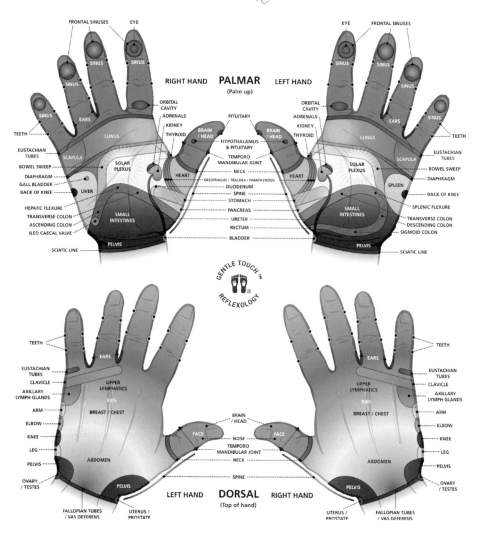

RIGHT HAND **PALMAR** **LEFT HAND**
(Palm up)

Right Hand labels (left to right, top to bottom): FRONTAL SINUSES, EYE, SINUS, SINUS, SINUS, SINUS, EARS, TEETH, LUNGS, EUSTACHIAN TUBES, SCAPULA, BOWEL SWEEP, DIAPHRAGM, GALL BLADDER, BACK OF KNEE, LIVER, HEPATIC FLEXURE, TRANSVERSE COLON, ASCENDING COLON, ILEO CAECAL VALVE, SMALL INTESTINES, SOLAR PLEXUS, PELVIS, SCIATIC LINE

Center labels: ORBITAL CAVITY, ADRENALS, KIDNEY, THYROID, BRAIN / HEAD, PITUITARY, HYPOTHALAMUS & PITUITARY, TEMPORO MANDIBULAR JOINT, NECK, HEART, OESOPHAGUS / TRACHEA / PARATHYROIDS, DUODENUM, SPINE, STOMACH, PANCREAS, URETER, RECTUM, BLADDER

Left Hand labels: EYE, FRONTAL SINUSES, SINUS, SINUS, SINUS, SINUS, EARS, TEETH, LUNGS, EUSTACHIAN TUBES, SCAPULA, BOWEL SWEEP, DIAPHRAGM, SPLEEN, BACK OF KNEE, SOLAR PLEXUS, SPLENIC FLEXURE, TRANSVERSE COLON, DESCENDING COLON, SIGMOID COLON, SMALL INTESTINES, PELVIS, SCIATIC LINE

GENTLE TOUCH™ REFLEXOLOGY®

LEFT HAND **DORSAL** **RIGHT HAND**
(Top of hand)

Left Hand (dorsal) labels: TEETH, EARS, EUSTACHIAN TUBES, CLAVICLE, AXILLARY LYMPH GLANDS, ARM, ELBOW, KNEE, LEG, PELVIS, OVARY / TESTES, UPPER LYMPHATICS, RIBS, BREAST / CHEST, ABDOMEN, PELVIS, FALLOPIAN TUBES / VAS DEFERENS, UTERUS / PROSTATE

Center (dorsal) labels: BRAIN / HEAD, FACE, NOSE, TEMPORO MANDIBULAR JOINT, NECK, SPINE

Right Hand (dorsal) labels: TEETH, EARS, EUSTACHIAN TUBES, CLAVICLE, AXILLARY LYMPH GLANDS, ARM, ELBOW, KNEE, LEG, PELVIS, OVARY / TESTES, UPPER LYMPHATICS, RIBS, BREAST / CHEST, ABDOMEN, PELVIS, UTERUS / PROSTATE, FALLOPIAN TUBES / VAS DEFERENS

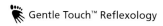

Gentle Touch™ Reflexology

Index

Rejection 20
Relax 10, 31, 38, 39, 53, 81
Reproductive Organs 113, 114
Respecting 20
Respiratory Systems 81
Responses and Reactions 29
Responsibilities 113
Rest and Relaxation 103, 110
Ribs 53, 126
Ridges 61
Right Hand 126
Right Hand Side 41, 126
Right Sole 124
Rogue 'Tummy' Ache 92
Role of a Reflexology Practioner 89
Root / Base Chakra 114, 115
Root Cause 26
Run 23

S

Sacral 113, 114, 115, 123
Sacrum Spine 124
Safety 18
Sanskrit 112
Scalp 114
Scanning 21
Scapula 124, 126
School 23, 26, 31, 40
Sciatic 75, 124, 126
Scope of the Treatment 25
Sedate 49
Self Confidence 10
Self Esteem 10
Self Expression 113
Self Preservation 113
Senate Document number 264, 105
Senses 114
Sensitive 60, 61
Sensory 88
Seriously 13
Serotonin 86
Sha Line 108
Shampoos 106
Shape 21
Shape of the Toes 22
Sharp 61
Shocks 56
Shoes 21, 65, 97, 99, 100
Shoulder 26, 54, 55, 114, 113, 115
Shower Gel 106
Shower Rooms 100
Showers 96
Sick 17, 20, 25, 115
Sigmoid Colon 72, 73, 78, 114, 124, 126
Signed Consent 22
Sinus 47, 48, 81, 86, 113, 124, 126
Size of Baby or Child's Feet 35
Skelatal 40, 45, 56, 114
Skin 21, 22, 93, 106, 115
Skull 45, 61, 124
Sleep 10, 60, 81, 86, 107, 108
Sleeping Area 108

Splenic Flexure 72
Small Intestine 71, 74, 75, 85, 87, 115, 124, 126
Smelly Feet 97
Smile 16, 38
Snoring 92
Social Interaction 88
Socks 21, 65, 97, 99, 100
Sodium Laureth Sulphate (SLES) 106
Sodium Lauryl Sulphate (SLS) 106
Soft Tissue Damage 55
Solar Plexus 40, 42, 53, 67, 71, 76, 82, 83, 84, 85, 86, 87, 113, 114, 115, 122, 124, 126
Solar Plexus Chakra 114
Sore Throat 64
Soul Chakra 115
Special Needs 13, 88
Special Occasions 31
Spinal Reflexes 60
Spine 42, 59, 114, 114, 122, 124, 126
Spiritual Centre 113
Spleen 73, 114, 124, 126
Splenic Flexure 73, 124, 126
Sports Centre 96
Stages of Progess 41
Stagnated 49
Start of the Treatment 37
Sternum 114
Steroids 93
Stomach 82, 84, 87, 115, 124, 126
Stomach Aches 37
Stress 53, 89
Stress Buster 53
Stress Indicators 114
Stressed 62
Subtle 22, 40, 55, 65
Success Tips for Reflexology 15
Suffering 16
Sugar 115
Supermarkets 105
Supplementation 105
Sweat Glands 97
Sweetness 115
Swimming Baths 96
Switzerland 106
Symptoms 28

T

Talking 103, 110
Tea Tree Oil 99
Teenagers / Teens 56, 66
Teeth 46, 47, 50, 87, 114, 124, 126
Teething 81, 86, 87
Telephone Numbers 24
Temperature 17, 21
Temporomandibular Joint (TMJ) 45, 49, 59, 71, 84, 85, 86, 87, 124, 126
Temporal Region 45
Tension 17, 56, 114
Testes 76, 126
Texture 21, 22, 53
The Cuddle 78
Therapeutic Touch 88
Thoracic Spine 123, 124, 126

Reflexology Reminders

Enjoy giving the treatments and stay relaxed

Pay attention to your own comfort and health

Work very lightly and gently

Always follow your intuition or "gut instincts"

Take your time

Work for as long as both the practitioner and child are open, receptive or are enjoying it

Where Do You Go From Here?

I hope that you have enjoyed the book and that it has developed your perception of what is possible. If you would like to take it further there are a number of options available to you:

- Arrange an appointment with Sue Ricks Clinic or a qualified reflexologist that specialises in working with babies and children

- Undertake a professional reflexology training or further advanced courses

Many Courses, tutorials and internet based learning opportunities are detailed on the web site www.suericks.com

Further Information

Organisations

Association of Reflexologists www.aor.org.uk
British Register of Complementary Practitioners www.icnm.org.uk
Federation of Holistic Therapists www.fht.org.uk
Reflexology Association of America www.reflexology-usa.org
Reflexology Association of Australia www.reflexology.org.au

Courses

Many Courses, tutorials and internet based learning opportunities are detailed on the web site www.suericks.com

Including Gentle Touch™ Reflexology
Advanced reflexology courses
Energy and chakra courses
Life Skills
Book writing

Please contact suericks@suericks.com for more information on registered Gentle Touch™ Reflexology teachers.

Photos

Angelic Group www.angelicphoto.co.uk
Element One www.e1photo.co.uk
David Ricks
Sue Ricks

Contact

Sue Ricks School of Complementary Therapies,
Clinic - Leicestershire UK
Tel: +44 (0)1509 214 373
Email: suericks@suericks.com
Web: www.suericks.com
Facebook: facebook.com/Sue.Ricks.UK/